# Electrocardiography

by Cheryl Passanisi, RN, MS

## *Clinical Allied Healthcare Series*

Kay Stevens, RN, MA
Series Editor

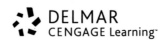
DELMAR
CENGAGE Learning

Australia • Brazil • Japan • Korea • Mexico • Singapore • Spain • United Kingdom • United States

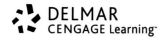

**Electrocardiography**
**Cheryl Passanisi**

Series Editor and Executive Director:
  Kay Stevens

Project Coordinator: Valerie L. Harris

Editors: William C. Klein, Valerie L. Harris

Illustrators: William C. Klein, Alan J. Borie,
  Valerie L. Harris

Additional Graphics obtained from the
LifeART™ Collections from Lippincott
Williams & Wilkins, Cleveland, OH.

Cover Design: Harris Graphics

For product information and technology assistance, contact us at
**Cengage Learning Customer & Sales Support, 1-800-354-9706**

For permission to use material from this text or product,
submit all requests online at **www.cengage.com/permissions**
Further permissions questions can be emailed to
**permissionrequest@cengage.com**

Library of Congress Control Number: 00-108728

ISBN-13: 978-0-89262-435-5

ISBN-10: 0-89262-435-3

**Delmar**
Executive Woods
5 Maxwell Drive
Clifton Park, NY 12065
USA

Cengage Learning is a leading provider of customized learning solutions with
office locations around the globe, including Singapore, the United Kingdom,
Australia, Mexico, Brazil, and Japan. Locate your local office at
**www.cengage.com/global**

Cengage Learning products are represented in Canada by Nelson Education, Ltd.

To learn more about Delmar, visit **www.cengage.com/delmar**

Purchase any of our products at your local bookstore or at our preferred online
store **www.cengagebrain.com**

Printed in the United States of America
13 14 15 16 17     22 21 20 19 18

# Dedication

To all my patients who have patience with me and provide new and exciting learning experiences every day. Thanks!

# Contents

# Acknowledgements

The author would like to thank everyone who graciously contributed to the formation of this text. The contributions of the following are particularly appreciated.

Kay Stevens, RN, MA, Series Editor and Valerie Harris, Project Coordinator, for keeping me on my toes, always honing and perfecting.

Debra Garber, RN, BSN, MICN, EMT-P, of Carson-Tahoe Hospital in Carson City, Nevada and Julie Caley, RN, BSN, of the Shasta Trinity Regional Occupational Program in Redding, California for their meticulous reviews of the text.

Phyllis Casparian, Administrator of Cardiology Specialists of Orange County in Santa Ana, California for her assistance in obtaining Holter monitor photographs.

Malcolm Pond, MD, Chiayu Chen, MD, and the staff at Riverside Cardiology Associates in Riverside, California for their assistance in obtaining 12-Lead ECG photographs.

Jim Clover, ATC, PTA of the S.P.O.R.T. Clinic in Riverside, California for his assistance in obtaining 12-Lead ECG photographs.

# Introduction

To work in the medical field is to make a real contribution to your fellow man. This is a career that will ask much of your mind and heart and give much in return. The satisfaction gained from calming a frightened child or brightening the day of a lonely patient will enrich you. The pride felt will be lasting when your observations and skills someday help to save a patient's life. This is a career where you can really make a difference!

Some of you have already made a decision to seek a career in some area of healthcare. Some of you are just exploring your options. Everything you learn will build a foundation of skills and knowledge, so learn well. Become competent in everything you are taught along the way and be your own task master. We all must be responsible for our own education. If at some point you discover you didn't learn a skill well enough, go back and practice until you do. Remember, some day a patient's life may depend on you and your mastery of what you are taught.

Today's healthcare industry places many demands on care givers. We must keep costs down, document everything we do, and have more knowledge and skills than ever before because of new technology. This textbook series was designed to help you build a sound foundation of knowledge and provide many opportunities for cross-training. This core textbook contains the skills and information we feel is common to all students. Each of the other textbooks provide training for a specific job title. The more you can learn, the better. Always remember, however, to practice the art, the science, and the SPIRIT of your new career. Good luck!

Kay Stevens, RN, MA
Series Editor

# Contributors

### About the Author

Cheryl Passanisi, RN, MS has many years of experience as a cardiovascular nurse. She earned a BS in nursing from California State University, Long Beach. At the University of California, San Francisco, Ms. Passanisi received an MS in the Cardiovascular Clinical Nurse Specialist program. She has worked in the coronary care unit (CCU), cardiovascular intensive care, emergency department, telemetry/stepdown units, as well as cardiac rehabilitation. Ms. Passanisi has special interests in patient education and compliance issues. She has studied psychology and the psychological factors in cardiovascular disease and the recovery process. Ms. Passanisi currently works as an assistant nurse manager of an intermediate cardiac care unit.

### About the Series Editor

Kay Stevens, RN, MA conceived this textbook series, and recruited and coordinated the authors in the development of each of their texts. She is the author of *Being a Health Unit Coordinator,* and the editor of a Medical-Clerical Textbook Series for Brady. Before entering education, she worked in medical/surgical and critical care nursing and in the inservice department as a clinical instructor.

Formerly a Professional Development Contract Consultant for special projects and curriculum development for the California Department of Education, Professor Stevens has also served as chairperson of the California Health Careers Statewide Advisory Committee, and been a Master Trainer for Health Careers Teacher Training through California Polytechnic University of Pomona. She also is a founding member of the National Association of Health Unit Coordinators. Professor Stevens is currently Program Coordinator of the Medical Assistant Program at Saddleback College in Mission Viejo, California, and operates her consulting business, Achiever's Development Enterprises.

# Editor's Note

I would like to take this opportunity to thank the authors of this series. Their dedication and sense of mission made it a joy to work on this challenging project. I particularly wish to thank and congratulate the author of this text, Cheryl Passanisi, for her professionalism and hard work on this book.

I would also like to express my sincere gratitude to the staff of Career Publishing, Inc. and most especially Valerie Harris for her professional and talented assistance throughout. I also would like to express my appreciation to Harold Haase, Publisher, for his enthusiasm for this project and for his humanistic approach to education.

Kay Stevens, RN, MA
Series Editor

## Chapter One
# Introduction to the Role

## *Objectives*

After completing this chapter, you should be able to
do the following:

1. Define and correctly spell each of the key terms.

2. Describe the role and responsibilities of the ECG technician.

3. List the qualities and attributes an ECG technician should have.

4. Describe the work environment of an ECG technician.

# Key Terms

- cardiology
- cardiovascular
- conflict resolution
- electrocardiogram (ECG, EKG)

- electrocardiograph
- Patient's Bill of Rights
- prioritize

# Introduction

**electrocardiograph:**
a machine used to record the electrical activity of the heart.

**electrocardiogram:**
ECG or EKG; a recording of the electrical activity of the heart. A recording made by an electrocardiograph.

**cardiovascular:**
of or relating to the heart and blood vessels.

The **electrocardiograph** technician, or **ECG** tech, is an important member of the healthcare team. The role of the ECG tech is to assist the physicians and nurses in collecting information about a patient's heart using an electrocardiograph. The **electrocardiogram**, or ECG, is a recording of the electrical impulses that produce the heartbeats, or contractions, of the heart. The ECG shows if the heart muscle is damaged, or if it is beating irregularly. The ECG is an important diagnostic tool in determining the health and function of the **cardiovascular** system.

The information the ECG technician records helps to determine the diagnosis and treatment plan for the patient. This information, in the form of the ECG, becomes part of the patient's permanent health record. Therefore, completeness and accuracy is essential in performing an ECG.

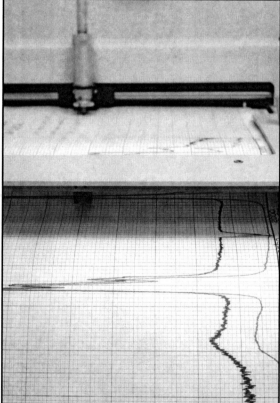

*Figure 1-1: An electrocardiograph is used to collect information about a patient's heart function.*

# The Role and Responsibilities of the ECG Technician

ECG technicians work in hospitals, clinics, and physician's offices. Their duties include assisting doctors and nurses with cardiac tests such as ECGs and treadmill stress tests, as well as taking care of the equipment used in obtaining these tests. The technician usually explains the procedure to the patient and often prepares the patient for the procedure by connecting the patient to the ECG machine. The technician is also responsible for the quality of the ECG recording. High quality is assured by completely explaining the procedure to the patient, so he or she can cooperate fully. The quality is also assured by reporting equipment malfunctions to the engineers who are responsible for repairing the equipment.

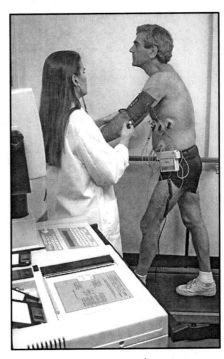

When ECG technicians work in hospitals, they usually take the ECG machine to the patient's room to perform the ECG. Often the patient is too sick to get out of bed, and the technician must help the patient get into the proper position. Many times the technician must check with the charge nurse for further instructions. For instance, the patient may be attached to tubes or devices that must be handled with special care. In this case, the nurse would assist the technician in hooking up the ECG machine, or give the technician special instructions.

*Figure 1-2: ECG technicians assist with stress tests, which measure the ability of a patient's heart to respond to the stress of exercise.*

Frequently, the patient or family members are frightened of tests that are performed in hospital settings. In these instances, it is vital for the technician to have good communication skills. Communicating with patients or family members of patients and explaining the procedure in terms they can understand is important because it helps to calm the anxious patient and helps the patient to cooperate and relax.

Communicating effectively with nurses and other healthcare workers is also important. Learning the basic terminology used in this field is an important part of effective communication with coworkers. Communication will also be enhanced by understanding something about the heart and heart disease. You will have an opportunity to learn more about these topics in later chapters.

The ECG technician may also work in a physician's office or in a clinic setting. In these settings, the patients usually will have an appointment and come to an office where the technician is located. Patients in a clinic or office are called "outpatients" and usually are not as sick as patients in the hospital. Outpatients still need a clear explanation of the procedure and may require special consideration. For example, the technician must be on the alert for patient problems that might present challenges during the procedure, such as patients who have difficulty hearing or who have arthritis.

**Patient's Bill of Rights:** a document that identifies the basic rights of all patients.

In all settings, the technician must demonstrate respect for the patient and maintain confidentiality of the patient's treatment records. This means that the technician cannot share any information about patients with anyone except healthcare workers directly involved in the care of the patient. All health centers have strict rules regarding confidentiality. Most states and healthcare institutions have established a document called the **Patient's Bill of Rights**. Confidentiality and rights to privacy are important elements in the Patient's Bill of Rights. There should be no gossiping about patients or discussion of patient problems outside of the workplace. Respect for patients is also a key element of the Patient's Bill of Rights.

ECG technicians may be assigned different titles or names at various institutions, but the roles and responsibilities are similar. Other duties that may be assigned include filing paperwork, answering phones, or delivering messages.

# Patient's Bill of Rights

1. The patient has a right to considerate and respectful care.

2. Patients have the right to obtain from their physician complete current information concerning their diagnosis, treatment and prognosis in terms they can be reasonably expected to understand.

3. An informed consent should include knowledge of the proposed procedure, along with its risks and probable duration of incapacitation. In addition, the patient has a right to information regarding medically significant alternatives.

4. The patient has the right to refuse treatment to the extent permitted by law, and to be informed of the medical consequences of his action.

5. Case discussion, consultation, examination, and treatment should be conducted discretely. Those not directly involved must have the patient's permission to be present.

6. The patient has the right to expect that all communication and records pertaining to his care should be treated as confidential.

7. The patient has the right to expect the hospital to make a reasonable response to his request for services. The hospital must provide evaluation, service, and referral as indicated by the urgency of the case.

8. The patient has the right to obtain information as to any relationship of his hospital to other healthcare and educational institutions, insofar as his care is concerned. The patient has the right to obtain information as to the existence of any professional relationships among individuals, by name, who are treating him.

9. The patient has the right to be advised if the hospital proposes to engage in or perform human experimentation affecting his care or treatment. The patient has the right to refuse to participate in such research projects.

10. The patient has the right to expect reasonable continuity of care.

11. The patient has the right to examine and receive an explanation of his bill regardless of the source of payment.

12. The patient has the right to know what hospital rules and regulations apply to his conduct as a patient.

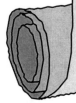

*Figure 1-3: A Patient's Bill of Rights*

# Requirements and Attributes of the ECG Technician

**cardiology:** the medical specialty which is the study of the heart and diseases of the heart.

Those interested in becoming an ECG technician should have graduated from high school or obtained an equivalent diploma. Basic math and reasoning skills are important, as is an interest in the field of healthcare, particularly **cardiology**. Anatomy and physiology classes are helpful, but not necessary. In addition, ECG technicians should be interested in working in a technical environment. They will be responsible for handling specialized equipment that requires meticulous care and strict operating procedures.

It's worth emphasizing that strong communications skills are crucial in this field. Communication with doctors, nurses, other technicians, and patients should be clear and concise. This requires some knowledge of healthcare terminology as well as good speaking and writing skills. The ability to convey accurate instructions to patients compassionately is the technician's most valuable asset.

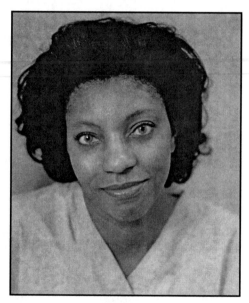

*Figure 1-4: Strong math skills, a good bedside manner, and the ability to communicate clearly are some of the important traits an ECG technician should possess.*

ECG technicians should enjoy working with people. Caring for patients with compassion and understanding is essential. Patients often will trust a healthcare worker based on the care, respect, and concern that is shown to them — not on the individual's skill and training. This overall attitude is known as the healthcare worker's "bedside manner." Your attitude, mannerisms, and tone of voice communicate the degree of genuine interest you have in the patient.

As an ECG technician, you will need cooperation from the patient in order to complete tests and procedures. If the patient does not sense sincere concern on your part, it will be difficult to enlist his or her cooperation and win the patient's trust. Without patient cooperation and trust, completion of tests and procedures is difficult.

A patient's disease and the uncertainty it causes can create anxiety for the patient. This anxiety can also be referred to as the "stress" of an illness. Everyone deals with stress in different ways. Therefore, the technician must be sensitive to the emotional state of the patient. A behavior that seems rude may actually be a coping mechanism for the patient, a way the patient can maintain a sense of self-esteem and regain control in his or her life. For example, when a patient is uncooperative, it may mean that he or she is anxious or afraid. When you encounter a situation like this, it is important to realize that the patient may be directing his or her anger AT you, but he or she is not angry WITH you. This type of behavior is called "displacement" or "projection." Informed healthcare workers learn how to identify this behavior and avoid taking it personally.

The best way to deal with patient anxiety and anger is through communication and education. Take the time to explain procedures and disease processes to your patients. Direct patients to doctors or nurses for more complete explanations if you do not have the information the patients are seeking. You may not know or have all the answers, but you can respond to the patient's questions to the best of your ability. This helps the patient to feel at ease and establish a sense of trust with you, the technician. However, you must never attempt to give a diagnosis (what is wrong with the patient), a prognosis (what the outcome of the patient's condition will be), or prescribe treatment. That is the doctor's job — not yours.

Flexibility is another essential characteristic of a healthcare worker. The medical field is filled with many regulations, complicated procedures, and a seemingly rigid chain of command. Many of these rules are important to ensure the safety and quality of patient care. But frequently the expected flow of activity is overridden in order to accommodate last-minute additions to the schedule, emergencies, equipment failures, or personnel problems (sick calls, etc.). Following a pre-planned schedule while addressing emergencies requires problem-solving skills. One of the most valuable problem-solving skills a person can possess is **conflict resolution**; it requires effective communication skills and the ability to compromise.

**conflict resolution:** solving problems created by opposing ideas or interests through the use of effective communication and compromise.

Conflict resolution involves the following steps:

1. Identify the problem.

2. Seek input from another person to get his or her point of view.

3. Both parties offer compromise.

For example, let's say that you have a patient who is uncooperative. He gets agitated when lying down and will not listen to your instructions.

Use the steps to solve the problem:

1.  Identify the problem.
    Example: Tell the nurse that a patient is uncooperative.

2.  Seek input from another person to get his or her point of view.
    Example: Allow the nurse to provide input. (eg, "The patient may be uncooperative because he gets short of breath when lying flat.")

3.  Both parties offer compromise.
    Example: The nurse may offer to assure the patient who is anxious and supply oxygen if necessary. The technician may offer to find an extra pillow to raise the patient's head slightly.

Or, imagine that a coworker has called in sick and you are unable to handle all of the ECG patients by yourself.

1.  Identify the problem.
    Example: Tell the nurse that you have more ECGs to do than can be accomplished during the given time frame.

2.  Seek input from another person to get his or her point of view.
    Example: Allow the nurse to provide input. (eg, "These are the patients who are in the greatest need of an ECG.")

3.  Both parties offer compromise.
    Example: The nurse may offer to do the most critical ECGs to free the technician to do the routine tests. The technician may offer to go to lunch 30 minutes later than scheduled in order to accommodate the volume of patients. Or, the nurse could call the supervisor to assist the technician and the technician could call a technician from another part of the hospital to see if he or she can assist with the increased volume of patients.

One very important problem-solving skill is the ability to **prioritize**. Prioritizing means arranging tasks in order of importance. Guidelines for prioritizing revolve around the patients. Remember, the sickest patient is always the

priority. You may not have the expertise to identify the most urgent patient situation. In that case, ask for guidance from the nurse, supervisor, or senior technician. For example, a patient experiencing chest pain would need an ECG immediately, whereas a patient requiring an ECG for a routine physical could wait awhile.

**prioritize:**
to arrange tasks
in order of
importance.

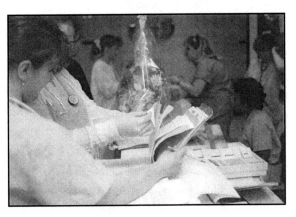

Figure 1-5: A nurse or senior technician can provide valuable assistance in determining which patients must be attended to first.

Another example of prioritizing would be if a patient has a language barrier. If the interpreter can only be available during a specified period of time, it is necessary to perform the ECG accordingly. It may be that a family member is interpreting, but must leave soon. Then, this ECG has priority. Or, maybe an interpreter will not be available until later; then, the ECG may be postponed. It is always better to be able to explain the procedure prior to the test, as this reduces the patient's anxiety. The exception, of course, would be if the patient is experiencing pain.

A coworker may call in sick, making it necessary for you to take on his or her assignments in addition to your own. If this is not physically possible, you may have to review the assignments with the supervisor and prioritize the patient list. Some patients may need to be rescheduled, or additional workers may need to be called in to help.

Equipment malfunctions may also make schedule adjustments necessary. These adjustments might include sharing equipment with another department, using backup equipment, and/or rescheduling procedures.

When patients require tests, it is necessary for the healthcare worker to follow a certain routine. Normally the technician checks the doctor's written order, confirms the patient's identity, and explains the procedure. However, if the patient is critical, then the technician may have to rely on a verbal order from the nurse or physician. You may also have to rely on the nurse's or physician's identification of the patient, and you may not have time to provide explanations to the patient. If this is the case, you will have to make written confirmations when the crisis has passed.

## Thinking It Through...

Imagine that you are an ECG technician in a busy clinic. Your schedule is booked solid with procedures. A doctor interrupts you just before you begin recording a routine ECG. He wants you to get an ECG on a patient in another room. The other ECG technician has called in sick, so there is no one else to help get the additional ECG. Before he is finished talking with you, a nurse interrupts the conversation to say that a patient has fainted down the hall, and an ECG is needed immediately.

1. How do you prioritize the many tasks that are requested of you?

2. What do you say to the doctor? What do you say to the nurse? What do you say to the patient who is waiting to have the routine ECG?

3. What are your conflict resolution strategies?

4. As you are playing the role of the ECG technician, do you feel pressured? Do you feel anxious? How do you deal with the stress?

Good communication skills, behavior management skills, flexibility, compassion, and time management skills are important qualities that successful workers in the healthcare field must acquire or possess. Physically, healthcare workers can accomplish only a certain amount in a given time frame. Working together as a team allows healthcare personnel to complete required work while focusing on quality patient care.

As an ECG technician it also is important to recognize the need for continuing education. Procedures, technology, and equipment change constantly in the healthcare field. You must be willing to expand your knowledge and keep up-to-date on new technologies and methods. Updating your knowledge increases the quality of care you provide to patients.

# The Stress Factor

As an ECG technician, you will find that your job can be exciting and challenging. But, as a member of the healthcare team, you will also encounter stressful situations. Organizing busy schedules, handling emergencies, dealing with anxious patients, and responding to demands from doctors and nurses can be frustrating.

Proper nutrition, adequate sleep, and regular exercise can help in managing stress. Knowing your limits as a healthcare worker is also important. Asking for help with tasks may also assist you in relieving stress. Do not be concerned that a request for help will reflect negatively on your capabilities. Instead, it indicates your commitment to quality patient care. You can also ask your friends and colleagues how they deal with stress. Their answers can give you additional ideas for managing stressful situations.

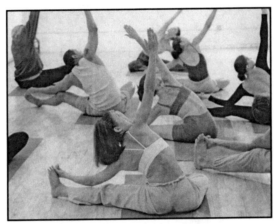

*Figure 1-6: Exercise is an effective way to reduce stress.*

# Chapter Summary

The ECG technician is a member of the allied healthcare team who assists physicians and nurses in collecting information about the heart. ECG technicians are trained to perform an ECG, which is a recording of the electrical activity of the heart. This information can be used to diagnose heart disease. Successful ECG technicians should enjoy working with people and technical equipment, possess strong communication skills, have the ability to prioritize and resolve conflicts, and never fail to demonstrate compassion.

Name_____

Date_____

# Student Enrichment Activities

**Complete the following statements.**

1. Three qualities that are valuable for an ECG technician to possess include:

   _____, _____, and _____.

2. A student considering a career as an ECG technician should be interested in

   _____, and especially in _____.

3. ECG technicians may be employed at _____, _____,

   and _____ _____.

4. _____ is a term refering to patients who are seen in a clinic or

   doctor's office.

5. The document that identifies the basic rights of all patients is called the

   _____ _____ _____ _____.

6. An ECG is an _____ _____ of the heart beat.

7. _____ _____ involves finding solutions to problems that

   may arise while performing the tasks of one's job, and compromise is a key to a

   successful outcome of those problems.

8. To accomplish more important tasks first and then, if time allows, to work on less

   important tasks is called _____.

9.  Three ways to help manage and control stress from your job are _____
    _____, _____ _____, and
    _____ _____.

**Complete the following exercises.**

10. Imagine that you are a patient who has come to see the doctor because you have
    been feeling tired lately and you experience chest pain whenever you mow the
    lawn or lift heavy objects. A longtime friend has recently died of a heart attack.
    You are afraid and nervous. The doctor has just ordered an ECG for you. You have
    never had this test before. What kind of questions will you have for the doctor?
    For the ECG technician? What kind of feelings are you experiencing? What kind
    of behavior do you expect from the healthcare workers assisting you? What kind
    of behavior would help to put you at ease? What kind of behavior would make
    you feel more anxious?

    _____

    _____

    _____

    _____

    _____

    _____

    _____

    _____

    _____

    _____

    _____

    _____

    _____

    _____

    _____

Name_____

Date_____


**11.** Imagine that you work in the busy emergency room of a large hospital. It has been a very hectic day. Many patients have been admitted to the emergency room, and you have to perform ECGs on most of them. The charge nurse requests that you do an ECG on a patient who has just been admitted for chest pain. You go into the room where the patient is waiting. He immediately starts to yell at you. He claims that he is in severe pain and wants something immediately for pain. He says that this is a very inefficient hospital, and he wants to leave and go to another hospital. What do you say to the patient? How do you attempt to calm him? What emotions do you imagine he is feeling? What emotions are you feeling? Should you call the patient's nurse or doctor? What do you tell the patient about why he needs to have an ECG? What should you say or not say to the patient about his sensation of pain?

_____

_____

_____

_____

_____

_____

_____

_____

_____

_____

_____

_____

_____

_____

_____

12. After thinking about these situations or enacting them in a classroom, what have you learned about yourself? What "people skills" do you already possess? Which skills do you need to improve? How do you react under stress?

_____

_____

_____

_____

_____

_____

_____

_____

_____

_____

_____

_____

_____

_____

**Use a separate sheet of paper to complete the following exercise.**

13. Locate the "help wanted" ads in the classified section of the newspaper. Find ads for ECG technicians. What are the requirements for these positions? What are the settings for these jobs? What other job titles sound similar to that of ECG technician? How many different titles can you identify? Write an essay that explains your qualifications for the job.

# Chapter Two
# Fundamental Concepts

## *Objectives*

After completing this chapter, you should be able to
do the following:

1. Define and correctly spell each of the key terms.

2. Explain the term, "risk factor," and list three cardiac risk factors.

3. Explain the diseases and conditions that may affect the heart.

4. List tests that are used to determine the presence of heart disease.

# Key Terms

- angina
- angiogram
- arrhythmia (or dysrhythmia)
- arteriosclerosis
- artery
- atherosclerosis

- cardiac
- coronary arteries
- heart catheterization
- ischemia
- myocardial infarction
- risk factors

# Introduction to the Cardiac Patient

**cardiac:**
pertaining to
the heart.

The word **cardiac** is used by health professionals when referring to the heart. Thus, cardiac patients have some kind of heart problem or disease. This chapter will help to familiarize you with the profile of a typical cardiac patient. The types of problems these patients experience and a summary of treatment options will be reviewed as well as some of the terms used by healthcare workers in the field of cardiology.

# Cardiac Risk Factors

**risk factors:**
conditions or
states that
increase the
likelihood of
developing a
particular
disease.

Risk factors are conditions or states that increase the likelihood of developing a particular disease. Cardiac **risk factors** are those conditions or states which significantly increase the probability of developing heart disease. It is important for you, as an ECG technician, to have an understanding of cardiac risk factors. Even if your time with patients is limited, you may be able to clarify information for them or direct them to healthcare professionals who can give them more complete information. Every contact with a patient is an opportunity to provide vital information to a potentially frightened or confused individual.

Some risk factors can be altered and others cannot. If a risk factor can be changed, it means that as the risk factor changes, the risk for heart disease also changes. The American Heart Association has launched efforts to educate the public on its ability to change certain risk factors and, thus, reduce the risk of heart disease.

## Heredity

Heredity is a risk factor that cannot be changed. We are each born with a set of genes that cannot be altered. If a family member develops heart disease, then first-degree relatives (siblings, children, parents) have a greater likelihood of developing heart disease. Researchers are still studying this factor. It is thought that a gene or a set of genes may exist that makes an individual **predisposed** (more likely) to developing certain diseases. This doesn't mean that if heart disease runs in the family, every member is assured of developing the disease, rather it means that there is a strong possibility of heart disease developing in some members of that family.

## Gender

Gender is another risk factor that cannot be altered. Men are more likely to develop coronary artery disease (CAD) than are pre-menopausal women. This predisposition is likely due to hormonal factors such as testosterone (male hormone) and estrogen (female hormone). However, as women age and estrogen secretion decreases (after menopause), the potential for developing CAD increases, making women as likely as men to develop the disease. Some studies have shown that in women who take estrogen replacement after menopause there is a decrease in the incidence of CAD. Other studies dispute this finding.

## Age

As we get older, we are more susceptible to the effects of CAD. This does not mean, however, that CAD is a part of the normal aging process. CAD is a distinct disease apart from the aging process. CAD develops over many years. Younger people with minimal narrowing of the arteries may not notice any symptoms. But as a person ages and the disease progresses, the narrowing becomes more severe and symptoms begin to appear. Aging causes blood vessels to lose elasticity, meaning that arteries have more difficulty dilating or expanding. Along with other physiological changes, this impaired ability to dilate results in decreased blood flow to tissues such as the heart muscle. Since blood carries oxygen to all of the body's tissues and cells, those changes may cause the symptoms of coronary artery disease (chest pain, shortness of breath, fatigue) to become more severe. The heart muscle weakens with age, decreasing the efficiency of its pumping action. The damage caused by a heart attack can also decrease the pumping action of the heart muscle. The effects of aging and damage from heart disease can result in severe impairment of heart function. With age, the heart is less able to compensate for damage caused by heart disease. CAD is a cumulative process, and as a person ages the fatty build up and the narrowing of the blood vessels progresses. Changes in the blood vessels and heart muscle during the aging process increase a person's susceptibility to the process of CAD.

## Hypertension

Hypertension is high blood pressure. This is a risk factor that CAN be changed. Research has shown that patients with high blood pressure have higher incidence of heart disease. When patients take their blood pressure medicine as prescribed, they may decrease their blood pressure, possibly improving their overall health, and thereby decreasing their risk for heart disease.

## Hyperlipidemia

Triglycerides and cholesterol are **lipids**, or fatty type substances. These are essential nutrients that we need to build body tissue and maintain the chemical functions of the body. High levels of triglycerides and cholesterol (hyperlipidemia) are associated with CAD. Exercise, diet, and medication are ways to decrease triglycerides and cholesterol.

## Diabetes

Diabetes is a disease in which the **glucose** (sugar) level in the blood is elevated. **Diabetics** (patients with diabetes) have a higher incidence of heart disease than people who do not have diabetes. Diabetics can decrease their risk for heart disease by keeping their blood sugar within the normal range through diet, exercise, and medication.

## Smoking

Smokers have a higher risk of heart disease than do nonsmokers. Chemicals in cigarette smoke can constrict blood vessels and increase the level of lipids in the blood. Those who stop smoking decrease their risk of developing heart disease. It is essential for smokers to understand that smoking is the single most important risk factor they can change. Programs that help people stop smoking are available in most communities.

## Diet

Diet is another risk factor that can be changed. Maintaining a low-fat diet that includes generous quantities of fresh fruits and vegetables, fish or fish oils, and whole grains is called a **heart healthy diet**. This type of diet eliminates or minimizes the amount of red meat that is eaten. The heart healthy diet has been shown to slow the rate of progression or even reverse heart disease. (Dean Ornish, 1990)

## Exercise

Physical activity and regular aerobic exercise are also beneficial for the heart. Exercise improves circulation and strengthens the heart muscle. Exercise can reduce lipid levels, lower blood pressure, and relieve stress.

## Obesity

A person who is obese is 20 - 30% or more over his or her ideal body weight. Obesity can contribute to high blood pressure and can cause increased strain on the heart. Often, it is a risk factor that may be changed.

## Stress

Many studies have shown that prolonged high levels of stress can contribute to heart disease and affect quality of life. This is a condition that affects everyone differently. It is important to know what situations are likely to cause stress in one's life, and it is equally important to have effective methods of dealing with that stress. These methods can include meditation, guided imagery, relaxation techniques, massage, and long walks.

# Disease Processes

Many diseases and conditions can affect the heart and the way it functions. The following is a brief description of the most common of them.

## Coronary Artery Disease (CAD)

**coronary arteries:**
blood vessels that bring oxygen rich blood to the heart muscle.

The **coronary arteries** supply oxygen rich blood to the heart muscle. Without this blood, the heart would be deprived of oxygen and would be unable to perform the pumping action that sends blood to other vital organs such as the brain. The disease process of **arteriosclerosis** causes a thickening of the **artery** wall and a loss of elasticity resulting in decreased blood flow through the artery. **Atherosclerosis** is a form of arteriosclerosis in which lipids or fats accumulate within the artery walls. As the fatty build-up progresses, blood flow through the artery is diminished. Atherosclerosis in the coronary arteries is called coronary artery disease (CAD) and results in decreased blood flow to the heart muscle. The lack of blood flow to the tissues of the heart results in a deficit of oxygen and nutrients. This condition, called **ischemia**, is one of the conditions that can be diagnosed by an ECG.

**arteriosclerosis:**
thickening and hardening of the arterial walls.

**artery:**
a blood vessel that carries highly oxygenated blood away from the heart to the tissues.

**atherosclerosis:**
narrowing of the arteries caused by fatty build-up within the artery wall and accompanied by a reduction in the artery's ability to dilate and constrict.

## Angina

Lack of blood flow to the heart will cause pain in the chest. Chest pain that is the result of ischemia often is referred to as **angina**. Angina may be the first symptom of heart disease, and it may be the initial reason that the patient seeks medical help. Any patient complaining of chest pain will need to have an ECG to assist in diagnosing the cause of the pain.

In the early stages of heart disease the patient may not notice any symptoms. As the disease progresses, however, the diminished blood flow will cause angina. Some patients may experience angina only during heavy exercise, when the heart muscle demands more oxygen and nutrients due to the increased work load. When a patient does not experience pain at rest, but does have pain with exercise, then a **treadmill stress test (TMST)** is ordered. During a TMST (also called a stress test, exercise ECG, or simply, treadmill), ischemia that occurs during exercise can be diagnosed. Patients who have advanced CAD may experience angina at rest as well as when exercising.

**ischemia:**
decreased blood flow to organs and tissues, such as the heart muscle, caused by the narrowing of the arteries.

**angina:**
chest pain caused by decreased blood flow to the heart.

It is important to keep in mind that all patients experience angina differently. Some will complain of a pressure in the chest frequently described as a "tightening band." Or, a patient may say, "It feels like an elephant sitting on my chest." Many patients will complain about a pain starting in the chest and radiating to the left arm or jaw. Others complain of a burning sensation, like indigestion, and may not believe that the pain is serious. Frequently, other symptoms such as **shortness of breath (SOB)**, anxiety, or light-headedness also occur.

## Myocardial Infarction (MI) or Heart Attack

Arteriosclerotic buildup in the arteries is thought to be the result of fatty deposits on the internal wall of the artery. Over time, calcium also is deposited onto the wall of the artery, making the artery rigid. This hardened deposit is called **plaque**. When the plaque forms in the wall of the artery, the wall is no longer smooth, but rough and uneven. This rough uneven surface increases the likelihood that blood clots will form in the artery. If a blood clot develops and totally occludes the artery, all blood flow through the artery is blocked. This condition results in a **myocardial infarction (MI)**, or **heart attack**. *Myocardial* is a term that refers to the heart muscle, and *infarction* means tissue death. So, *myocardial infarction* means death of heart muscle. During a complete block-age of an artery, the muscle tissue beyond the area of blockage will be deprived of oxygen and nutrients. (See Figure 2-1.) This means the tissue will die. An MI is a medical emergency. An ECG can aid in the diagnosis of an MI. Therefore, an ECG technician may be a part of the emergency team taking care of a patient with an MI.

**myocardial infarction:** a heart attack; the death of heart muscle caused by complete blockage of coronary arteries.

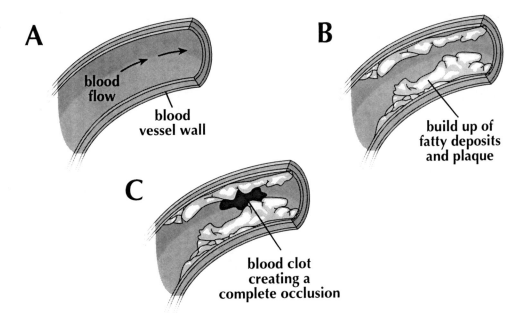

*From LifeART, Super Anatomy 2, Copyright 1998, Lippincott Williams & Wilkins.*

**A.** Normal vessel and normal blood flow. The inside of the blood vessel has a smooth surface.
**B.** Build-up of fatty acids and plaque create blockage and decreased blood flow, which can cause angina.
**C.** A blood clot can form, creating a complete blockage—the cause of a heart attack.

*Figure 2-1: Stages Leading to Blockage of a Blood Vessel*

During an MI, a patient may experience pain similar to angina, but the pain may be more severe and may last for a prolonged period of time. Other symptoms may include severe SOB, nausea and vomiting, anxiety, and diaphoresis (heavy sweating). The American Heart Association estimates that about 1.5 million people suffer from MIs each year. Of that number, about one third die before they even reach the hospital.

Often a patient will sense something is wrong, but will not want to admit that he or she may have a serious illness. The patient may postpone going to the doctor or hospital, thereby increasing the potential for serious complications and death. This behavior is called *denial*. Educational efforts aimed at informing the public about the signs and symptoms of heart disease and heart attacks and encouraging people to seek medical attention as soon as symptoms appear is a strategy that can save lives. There are many medicines and procedures that can increase the survival rate of cardiac patients and improve the quality of life after a heart attack. Prompt medical attention is the key to survival.

Some patients may have only minor symptoms of cardiac disease and attribute them to the flu or indigestion. In reality, they may indeed be having a heart attack and not realize it. If these patients survive, the cardiac event may be picked up on a future ECG. This is known as a *silent heart attack*.

## Cardiac Arrhythmia or Dysrhythmia

**arrhythmia:** dysrhythmia; an abnormal heart rhythm.

CAD, MI, and other cardiac diseases may cause disturbances in the rhythm of the heart. This disturbance is called cardiac **arrhythmia** or **dysrhythmia**. Usually the heart beats at regular intervals and provides a steady flow of blood to the rest of the body. When the heart beats irregularly, too fast, or too slow, the flow of blood may be reduced to the rest of the body, causing dizziness or fainting (syncope) episodes. Dysrhythmias can be either **chronic** (long term) or **acute** (immediate) problems. An ECG can help in the diagnosis of dysrhythmias.

# Diagnostic Tests and Treatment

Diagnostic tests and treatments can be **invasive** or **non-invasive**. Procedures, such as **heart catheterization** and open heart surgery, that require the insertion of instruments into the body are invasive. Procedures such as an ECG and an echocardiogram are non-invasive because they are performed on the body's surface.

## Heart Catheterization

The diagnostic test in which small tubes are passed into the heart chambers and the blood vessels around the heart is called heart catheterization. It is a technique used to gain access to the heart, take x-rays, and examine the heart valves and walls for abnormalities. This procedure is performed in a cardiac catheterization laboratory. The patient is awake during the procedure, but is given medication to help him or her relax.

## Angiogram

During a heart catheterization, dye is injected into the coronary arteries in order to detect blockages in the arteries. A moving x-ray or cine-angiogram is taken of the arteries injected with the dye. This diagnostic test is called an **angiogram**.

## Percutaneous Transluminal Coronary Angioplasty (PTCA)

A percutaneous transluminal coronary angioplasty (PTCA) is a treatment for blocked arteries that can be performed upon completion of an angiogram. While the patient is still on the operating table, a catheter with a balloon at the end is placed in the artery at the site of the blockage. As the balloon is inflated, it flattens the blockage and enlarges the diameter of the narrowed artery. This procedure increases blood flow to the heart, reduces ischemia to the heart tissue, and may prevent a myocardial infarction.

**heart catheterization:** the passage of tubes into the heart for the purpose of diagnosing cardiac disease.

**angiogram:** x-rays of arteries after the injection of dye which allows the visualization of the arteries and determination of blockages within the arteries.

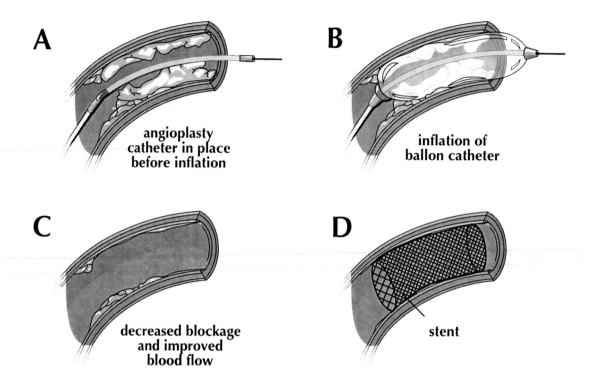

A
angioplasty
catheter in place
before inflation

B
inflation of
ballon catheter

C
decreased blockage
and improved
blood flow

D
stent

*From LifeART, Super Anatomy 2, Copyright 1998, Lippincott Williams & Wilkins.*

**A.** An angioplasty catheter is inserted at the site of the blockage.
**B.** The balloon at the tip of the catheter is inflated, compressing the blockage.
**C.** After the catheter is removed, the blockage is reduced and blood flow is improved.
**D.** A stent is a fine mesh made of metal, which can be placed in the artery to keep the blockage from returning.

*Figure 2-2: Angioplasty*

## Streptokinase and Tissue Plasminogen Activator (tPA)

Streptokinase and Tissue Plasminogen Activator (tPA) are medications called **thrombolytic agents**; they dissolve blood clots. They are administered to patients who are having a heart attack in order to dissolve the blood clot that is blocking the flow of blood to the heart tissues. If the medication is given in time, it can prevent permanent damage to the heart muscle. Streptokinase is less expensive than tPA, but tPA generally is preferred because it is specifically designed to attack the clot and creates fewer side effects, such as allergic reactions and excessive bleeding, than streptokinase. Cost and availability are the factors that determine which agent a given hospital will use. **Aspirin** also is given to thin the blood and prevent blood clots both during and after a heart attack.

## Coronary Artery Bypass Graft (CABG)

This procedure requires open heart surgery. When blockages in the heart cannot be successfully treated by a PTCA, then a patient may need to have surgery. In the CABG procedure, blood vessels from other parts of the body are removed (harvested). The harvested blood vessels are sewn directly into the aorta and then into the coronary artery beyond the blockage. These harvested blood vessels bypass the blockages, creating a free flow of blood to the deprived heart tissue. Thus, the heart muscle will get more oxygen and nutrients, and the patient should be able to live an active life without being limited by the frequent pain of angina.

## Cardioversion and Defibrillation

In a cardioversion, external electrical shocks are applied to a patient in order to correct a cardiac dysrhythmia—usually a rapid heart rate. The purpose of this procedure is to slow and regulate (convert the fast cardiac rhythm, ie, cardiovert) the heartbeat to a normal rate and rhythm. In contrast to cardioversion, defibrillation is another procedure whereby external electrical shocks are applied to a patient whose heart is beating in lethal dysrhythmia. Defibrillation actually stops the heart for a split second in order to allow the normal pacemaker of the heart to start again. The patient is unconscious, and has no pulse or blood pressure when this procedure is necessary.

## Implanted Cardiac Defibrillator (ICD)

This is a small defibrillator implanted into a patient's chest or abdomen that will automatically detect a dangerously fast heartbeat and defibrillate. This is often used as a last resort when medications have failed to regulate the heartbeat.

## Pacemaker

A pacemaker is a device used in patients whose heartbeat is too slow. The heartbeat may be slow because electrical conduction within the heart is **blocked**. The pacemaker ensures that a patient's heart rate will not go below a certain rate. Often, when taking an ECG on a patient with a pacemaker or ICD, the device will be visible as a raised disc under the skin in the upper chest or upper abdomen.

### Echocardiogram

An echocardiogram is a test that uses ultrasonic waves to obtain a picture of the chambers, valves, and walls of the heart. This test can also detect abnormalities of the heart valves and walls.

### Experimental Procedures

Laser and radiation techniques also are being perfected to use in treating coronary blockages. Lasers may be used in the future to remove or diminish blockages in the arteries, but this technique is still in development. Administering radiation to the inner wall of the artery may reduce buildup of blockages in the artery, but this is also still under investigation. In addition, ultrasound techniques are being used inside the vessel to give a more accurate picture of a blockage. This procedure is called intravascular ultrasound (IVUS).

# Chapter Summary

Heart disease affects many people and is the number one cause of death in the United States. Cardiac risk factors are conditions or behaviors that may increase the likelihood of developing heart disease. Some risk factors can be changed, while others cannot. Heart patients and others who want to prevent heart disease can examine their risk factors and often may change their behavior in order to decrease the likelihood of developing heart disease.

Angina is chest pain that is caused by diminished blood flow to the heart muscle. The decreased blood flow is due to atherosclerosis, the deposit of lipids (cholesterol and fatty acids) within the artery wall as well as the deposit of calcium, which causes the fatty build-up to harden and become a plaque. This causes blockage of the artery. When the condition becomes severe, myocardial infarction may occur. An MI occurs when an artery is completely blocked; it stops blood flow to that part of the heart, causing cell damage and tissue death. An MI can be fatal.

Diagnostic tests are designed to find evidence of blockage and decreased blood flow. An intervention can then be performed to decrease the blockage and restore blood flow before the patient experiences irreparable damage. New tests and interventions are being developed all the time. For example, researchers currently are trying to perfect the use of lasers to correct blockages in the coronary arteries.

Name_____

Date_____

# Student Enrichment Activities

**Match the term in Column A with the appropriate definition in Column B.**

## Column A

1. ___ angiogram

2. ___ ischemia

3. ___ coronary arteries

4. ___ angina

5. ___ arrhythmia

6. ___ MI

7. ___ echocardiogram

8. ___ CAD

9. ___ cardiac

## Column B

A. A heart test that uses ultrasound waves to obtain pictures of heart structures such as the valves and heart chambers.

B. Decreased blood flow to the tissue, resulting in decreased levels of oxygen and nutrients.

C. Blood vessels that bring oxygen-rich blood to the heart muscle.

D. Death of heart muscle tissue caused by blockages in the coronary arteries.

E. Chest pain caused by the decrease of blood flow to the heart muscle.

F. Relating to the heart.

G. Disturbance in the heart rhythm.

H. A procedure in which dye is injected into the coronary arteries and a moving x-ray is taken to detect blockages.

I. Heart disease caused by blockages in the coronary arteries.

**Complete the following statements.**

10. Patients with CAD may have diagnostic tests such as _____,
    _____, or _____.

11. Open-heart surgery is required for a _____.

12. A patient with CAD may experience symptoms such as _____,
    _____, and _____.

13. An undetected heart attack that is picked up on a future ECG is known as a
    _____ _____ _____.

14. Two terms for disturbances in the heart rhythm are _____ and
    _____.

15. CAD is caused by a _____ in the coronary artery.

16. The coronary arteries carry _____ and _____
    which are vital to the function of the heart muscle.

**Circle the correct answer.**

17. Risk factors that can be controlled or managed include all the following except:
    A. diet.
    B. sex.
    C. exercise.
    D. cholesterol level.
    E. hypertension.

Name_____

Date_____

## Define the following terms.

**18.** CABG: _____

_____

_____

**19.** PTCA:_____

_____

_____

**20.** defibrillation:_____

_____

_____

**21.** pacemaker: _____

_____

_____

**22.** risk factors: _____

_____

_____

# Chapter Three
# Cardiac Anatomy and Physiology

## *Objectives*

After completing this chapter, you should be able to
do the following:

1.  Define and correctly spell each of the key terms.

2.  Label the four chambers of the heart and describe the
    flow of blood through the heart.

3.  Identify the large blood vessels around the heart.

4.  Describe the significance of the electrical conduction
    system of the heart and the structures important to
    this system.

5.  Differentiate between the mechanical function and the
    electrical function of the heart.

6.  Define automaticity and its significance to heart function.

7.  Describe the importance of the heart as a pump and vital
    organ in the body.

## Key Terms

- aorta
- aortic valve
- atrioventricular node (AV node)
- atrium
- bundle branches
- bundle of His
- cellular membrane
- diastole
- electrolyte
- extracellular
- inferior vena cava
- intracellular

- mitral valve
- myocardium
- pericardial sac
- Purkinje fibers
- pulmonary arteries
- pulmonary veins
- pulmonic valve
- sinoatrial node (SA node)
- superior vena cava
- systole
- tricuspid valve
- ventricle

# Introduction to Anatomy and Physiology

Since the ECG technician is responsible for obtaining information about the heart, it is important to understand how the heart works. **Anatomy** refers to structure, and **physiology** refers to function. This chapter briefly describes cardiac anatomy and physiology—the structure and function of the heart.

# The Role of the Heart in the Body

The cells that make up the organs and tissues of the body require oxygen and nutrients to perform their specialized tasks. Cells also produce waste products that are toxic to the cells and need to be carried away. The heart is a pump that circulates the blood throughout the body to all the organs and tissues, a vital function. The oxygen is carried from the lungs to the tissues, and nutrients are brought from the intestinal tract to the tissues. Waste products are brought to the lungs, liver, and kidneys for detoxification or elimination. The movement of blood between the organs, the delivery of oxygen to the tissues, and the removal of waste products would not be possible without the pumping action of the heart.

Each minute, the heart pumps about five liters of blood. It beats at a rate of 60 to 100 times per minute. In a lifetime, the heart pumps millions of gallons of blood. The heart never stops to rest and never becomes fatigued the way a muscle in an arm or leg would become fatigued if it worked continuously. If the heart does stop, it is a medical emergency. This constant pumping is a tremendous task and would not be possible unless the heart was composed of special muscle cells and structures. Although this is a simplified description of the role of the heart, it reflects the importance of the heart and demonstrates how a diseased or damaged heart can threaten the health of the entire body.

## The Position of the Heart

The heart is a hollow, muscular organ about the size of a fist. It is located in the middle of the chest and tilts slightly to the left. The top of the heart is sometimes referred to as the base, and the bottom of the heart is referred to as the **apex**. The heart is stationed within the rib cage and is positioned between the right and left lungs. The rib cage is a rigid, bony structure that is designed to protect the vital organs enclosed within it, such as the heart, lungs, and the large blood vessels that carry blood toward and away from the heart. The **sternum** is a flat bone in the middle of the chest to which the individual ribs attach. The sternum, sometimes referred to as the breastbone, provides a protective function. The sternum and ribs are important landmarks used when examining the heart or performing an ECG. The heart usually lies between the 2nd and 5th **intercostal space** and extends from the edge of the right side of the sternum to the middle of the left side of the chest.

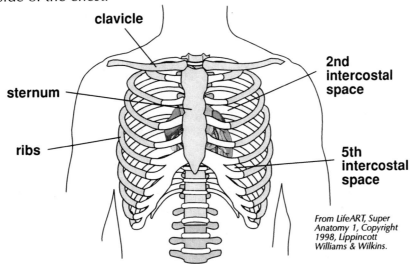

clavicle

sternum

ribs

2nd intercostal space

5th intercostal space

*From LifeART, Super Anatomy 1, Copyright 1998, Lippincott Williams & Wilkins.*

*Figure 3-1: Position of the Heart Within the Chest Cavity: Behind the Sternum, Between the 2nd and 5th Intercostal Spaces, Protected by the Rib Cage*

**myocardium:**
the heart muscle.

**atrium:**
one of the two top chambers of the heart, that receives blood from the large veins and then pumps blood into the lower chambers of the heart.

**superior vena cava:**
the main vein that drains blood from the upper part of the body into the right atrium of the heart.

**inferior vena cava:**
the main vein that drains blood from the lower part of the body into the right atrium of the heart.

**pulmonary vein:**
one of the two large vessels that returns oxygenated blood from the lungs to the left atrium.

**ventricle:**
one of the two large muscular pumping chambers of the heart located inferior to the atria.

**aorta:**
the large artery that receives blood from the left side of the heart and distributes the blood to the rest of the body.

# The Heart as a Muscle

The bulky muscular portion of the heart that performs the powerful pumping action is the **myocardium**. Each heartbeat is caused by the contraction of the heart muscle. With each heart beat, blood is ejected into the blood vessels. This action creates a pulse.

When viewed under a microscope, the cells that make up the heart muscle are all interconnected. This feature allows the electrical stimulation that causes contraction of the muscle to travel through the heart quickly and efficiently. The cardiac muscle cells are capable of contracting spontaneously, or without outside stimulation from nerves or chemicals. This ability to beat independently is called **automaticity**.

# Anatomical Structures of the Heart

## The Chambers

The heart muscle is divided into four areas called chambers. The heart is further divided into the right and left side. The **atria** are the small chambers at the top of the heart. The right **atrium** is on the right side of the heart and receives blood from the **superior vena cava** and the **inferior vena cava**. The left atrium is on the left side of the heart and receives oxygenated blood from the lungs by way of the **pulmonary veins**. The **ventricles** are large chambers in the lower part of the heart. The right ventricle is below the right atrium. The left ventricle is positioned below the left atrium. The left ventricle is much larger than the right because it has a bigger job to do. The right ventricle pumps blood to the system of vessels in the lungs via the pulmonary arteries, while the left ventricle pumps blood through the **aorta** to the rest of the body. The system of vessels that supplies the rest of the body is much larger than the system of vessels that supplies the lungs; therefore, the left ventricle has a larger volume (holds more blood in the chamber) and the muscle is thicker and stronger.

The heart is divided into right and left sides by a thick, muscular wall called the septum. The front wall of the heart lies against the left side of the rib cage. It is referred to as the **anterior wall** of the heart. The left ventricle is the major component of the anterior portion of the heart. The left wall of the heart is the lateral wall and faces the arm. The wall that faces the ribs in the back is the **posterior wall**. The wall that faces the lower half of the body is the **inferior wall**. The inferior wall is largely composed of the right ventricle, or the right side of the heart.

The 12-Lead ECG is capable of capturing a picture of these various "walls" of the heart. Abnormalities that reflect damage to one or more or these walls can be detected by an ECG.

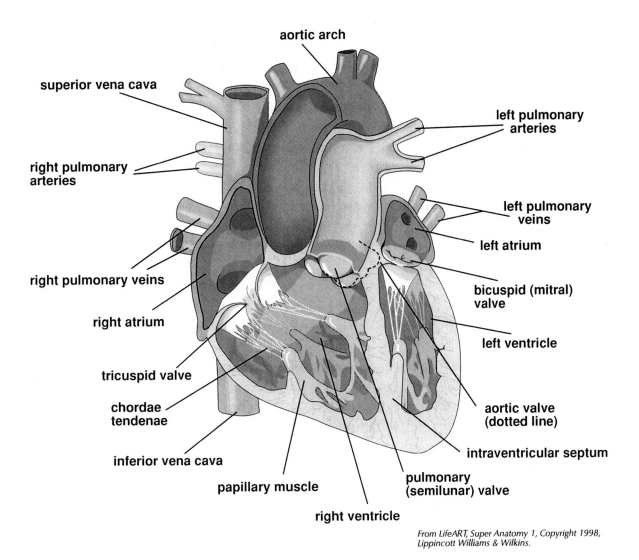

From LifeART, Super Anatomy 1, Copyright 1998,
Lippincott Williams & Wilkins.

*Figure 3-2: The Anatomical Structures of the Heart*

## The Valves

As the heart pumps, it is vital for the blood to flow through the heart in one direction. The forward movement of blood ensures that adequate amounts of blood will be delivered to the rest of the body. If a portion of the blood volume flows backwards, then the heart cannot get the blood out to the rest of the body. The forward movement of blood cannot happen without the presence of the heart **valves**, which are made of connective tissue, not muscle tissue. They are formed by leaflets that open in only one direction. As one heart chamber contracts, the build-up of pressure opens the valve and blood flows to the next chamber or vessel. As the next chamber contracts, it opens the valve located in front of the flow, but does not open the valve located behind the flow. This action demonstrates the one-way function of the valve that promotes the forward flow of blood. If the valves are damaged, blood can flow backward, causing major problems for the heart and lungs. For example, if the valves are not operating properly, then the heart may become enlarged because blood is not being expelled efficiently from a chamber. This makes the heart work harder to accomplish its task.

The **tricuspid valve** is positioned between the right atrium and right ventricle. It is called tricuspid because it has three cusps, or triangular leaflets. It prevents blood from flowing back into the right atrium from the right ventricle. The **pulmonic valve** lies between the right ventricle and the pulmonary artery. It prevents blood from flowing back into the right ventricle after it has been pumped into the pulmonary artery. The **bicuspid valve**, or **mitral valve**, is located between the left atrium and the left ventricle. It is called the bicuspid valve because it is formed from two cusps, or leaflets. This valve is commonly referred to as the "mitral valve" because it resembles the two cusps of a bishop's mitre. The mitral valve prevents the back flow of blood from the left ventricle into the left atrium. The **aortic valve** is located between the left ventricle and the aorta. It functions to maintain the forward motion of blood and prevents blood from re-entering the left ventricular chamber after the blood has been pumped into the aorta.

## The Pericardium

The fibrous membrane covering the entire heart is called the **pericardium**, or **pericardial sac**. This membrane contains a very small amount of fluid, called pericardial fluid, which prevents friction between the heart muscle and its surroundings as the walls of the heart move with each beat. The pericardial sac protects the heart from damage that may be caused by the friction of the heart's normal contractions and movements.

**tricuspid valve:** the three-cusp valve which controls the flow of blood between the right atrium and right ventricle.

**pulmonic valve:** the valve that is in the right ventricle and which separates the ventricle from the pulmonary artery.

**mitral valve:** the two-cusp valve separating the left atrium from the left ventricle.

**aortic valve:** the valve on the left side of the heart that opens to allow blood to flow from the left ventricle into the aorta.

**pericardial sac:** the fibrous covering which completely encloses and protects the heart.

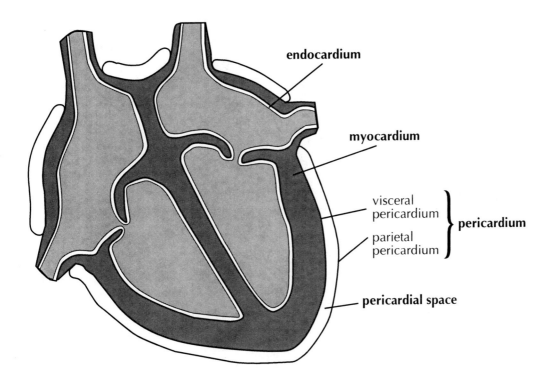

*Figure 3-3: The heart lies within the pericardial sac.*

# Circulation of Blood Through the Heart

The right atrium receives blood from other parts of the body through large veins called the **superior** and **inferior vena cava**. The superior vena cava collects blood from the upper part of the body, and the inferior vena cava collects blood from the lower part of the body. This blood comes from organs and tissues that have used up or depleted the oxygen from the blood cells. Blood that is depleted of oxygen and returns to the heart is called venous blood.

After the right atrium receives the venous blood from the superior vena cava and the inferior vena cava, the right atrium contracts, the tricuspid valve opens, and the oxygen-depleted blood enters the **right ventricle**. As the right ventricle contracts, the **pulmonic valve** opens and blood is ejected into the **pulmonary arteries**. The pulmonary arteries carry the blood to the lungs. In the lungs, the blood is able to exchange gases in the **alveoli**. The carbon dioxide that has built up in the blood is released through the lungs, and oxygen diffuses from the alveoli into the blood, enriching the blood with oxygen once again. The newly enriched blood then returns to the heart by way of the pulmonary veins that deliver the blood into the **left atrium**. As the left atrium contracts, the **mitral**

**pulmonary arteries:** large vessels that receive blood from the right ventricle and carry it to the lungs.

**valve** opens and the blood enters the **left ventricle**. The left ventricle is the main pumping chamber of the heart. It contracts and the **aortic valve** opens, delivering blood into the aorta. The aorta has many branches that deliver the oxygen-rich blood throughout the body.

The role of the heart is to keep the blood circulating. The right side of the heart delivers oxygen-depleted blood to the lungs where the blood cells are reoxygenated and returned to the heart. Then the left side of the heart delivers the oxygen-rich blood to the rest of the body.

## Blood Supply to the Heart

The heart muscle itself requires blood and oxygen. The **coronary arteries** branch off of the aorta and deliver blood to the heart muscle. These are the arteries that can become blocked with fatty build-up in coronary artery disease. When blood and the oxygen it carries can't get through to the heart muscle, ischemia or myocardial infarction (MI) can occur.

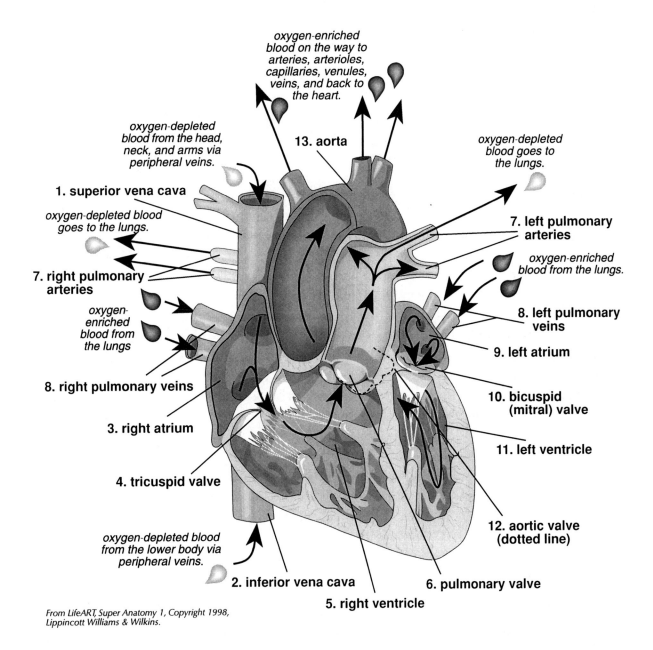

oxygen-enriched blood on the way to arteries, arterioles, capillaries, venules, veins, and back to the heart.

oxygen-depleted blood from the head, neck, and arms via peripheral veins.

13. aorta

1. superior vena cava

oxygen-depleted blood goes to the lungs.

7. right pulmonary arteries

oxygen-enriched blood from the lungs

8. right pulmonary veins

3. right atrium

4. tricuspid valve

oxygen-depleted blood from the lower body via peripheral veins.

oxygen-depleted blood goes to the lungs.

7. left pulmonary arteries

oxygen-enriched blood from the lungs.

8. left pulmonary veins

9. left atrium

10. bicuspid (mitral) valve

11. left ventricle

12. aortic valve (dotted line)

2. inferior vena cava

6. pulmonary valve

5. right ventricle

*From LifeART, Super Anatomy 1, Copyright 1998, Lippincott Williams & Wilkins.*

Blood returns to the heart through the inferior and superior vena cava, which empty into the right atrium. Blood flows through the tricuspid valve and into the right ventricle; then through the pulmonic valve and into the pulmonary arteries. From there, blood is delivered to the lungs in order to pick up oxygen and release carbon dioxide. The oxygen-rich blood then returns to the heart through the pulmonary veins and empties into the left atrium. Flowing through the mitral valve, the blood enters the left ventricle and proceeds through the aortic valve into the aorta and to the rest of the body.

*Figure 3-4: Flow of Blood Through the Heart*

# The Electrical Impulse in Heart Cells

The contraction of the heart muscle is a mechanical activity. But in order for the mechanical pumping to take place, an electrical impulse must stimulate, or initiate, the action. Both electrical activity and mechanical contraction occur at the cellular level. Electrical impulses are transmitted rapidly from cell to cell, causing the cells to contract. The end result is that the entire muscle contracts.

**electrolyte:** an ion or a small particle that is positively or negatively charged, such as sodium (Na+), potassium (K+), or chloride (Cl-).

In the body, electricity is conducted through the movement of **electrolytes** or **ions** across a semipermeable membrane. Ions are very small particles that have an electrical charge, either positive or negative. Sodium (Na+), potassium (K+), and calcium (Ca++) each carry a positive charge; chloride (Cl-) has a negative charge. As these ions move across a cellular membrane, an electrical impulse is initiated and sustained. Sodium and potassium are very important to this electrical activity in the body. Sodium is the most abundant electrolyte in the **extracellular** fluid, and potassium is the most abundant electrolyte in the **intracellular** fluid. Although both electrolytes are positively charged, the sodium ion carries a stronger charge than the potassium ion. This causes the **resting** (not contracting) cardiac cell to be positively charged on the outside of the cell membrane and negatively charged on the inside.

**extracellular:** fluid and particles outside of and surrounding the cell.

**intracellular:** within a cell.

In order for electrical conduction to occur, an exchange between ions or charged particles across the semi-permeable cellular membrane must take place. The three phases of electrical conduction are polarization, depolarization, and repolarization. Polarization is the resting state, meaning that there is a balance between the electrical charges on both sides of the cellular membrane and no movement of ions across the membrane occurs. During polarization, ions are poised on both sides of the membrane and ready for action.

**cellular membrane:** a layer of protein that surrounds a cell and keeps it separate from the surrounding fluid and cells.

As sodium and potassium trade places across the **cellular membrane**, they create a current, or wave, of electricity. This activity is known as **depolarization**. The electrical impulse travels throughout the heart and stimulates the mechanical contraction of the muscle during depolarization.

After depolarization, sodium and potassium again change places across the cellular membrane. Sodium moves out of the cell and potassium moves back into the cell. This process of the ions returning to their original places is called **repolarization**. The ions would not naturally move in this direction, so the mechanism of the *sodium pump* (the flow of electrons against their natural tendency) is used in the body to help repolarize the cells and tissues. When the cells are polarized, the cycle is then ready to begin again.

This description is a simplified version of the electrical stimulus in the cardiac muscle cell. It is important to remember that these events occur in fractions of a second. A polarization, depolarization, and repolarization event has to occur for each heartbeat, and a heartbeat occurs 60 to 100 times per minute. This indicates the rapidity of the electrolyte, or ion, movements across the cell membrane.

It is also crucial to understand that the events of polarization, depolarization, and repolarization are the very events that are being recorded by the ECG machine. Each of these events has a distinct tracing on the ECG. The actual waveforms will be described in later chapters. For now it is important to know that abnormalities recorded by the ECG are the result of disturbances in the polarization-repolarization cycle in the cells of the heart muscle. These disturbances can be the result of ischemia, injury, or infarction, which cause changes in the physiology of the heart muscle due to blood flow that is restricted or blocked. Electrolyte imbalances in the blood also cause changes in the electrical conduction and function of the heart muscle. These conditions can change the **morphology** (how the waveform looks, or its shape) and regularity of the waveform. Both morphology and regularity are factors that can be examined, measured, and analyzed on the ECG tracing.

# The Electrical Conduction System of the Heart

As stated earlier in this chapter, each cardiac cell is capable of automaticity (generating an electrical impulse). If each cell fired off electrical impulses at random, then the heart muscle would not be able to contract in a coordinated manner, and the effectiveness of the pumping action would be reduced or eliminated. Therefore, the heart needs a natural **pacemaker**. This pacemaker is called the **sinoatrial node**, or **SA node**. It is composed of specialized conductive tissue located high in the right atrium. The SA node generates electrical impulses at a rate of 60 to 100 times per minute. The electrical impulses that originate from the SA node create a waveform with a very specific morphology. This waveform is known as a **sinus rhythm**. It is described in detail in Chapter Eight.

**sinoatrial node:** (SA node) the natural pacemaker of the heart, located in the upper part of the right atrium.

The SA node has a rich supply of nerves that can influence the heart rate and the force of contraction. These nerves carry impulses from the brain to the heart via the central nervous system. Therefore, emotions and exercise will cause a change in heart rate, which enables the heart to adjust to the needs of the rest of the body.

**atrioventricular node:**
(AV node) special conductive tissue located in the lower right atrium that conducts electrical impulses from the atria to the ventricles.

**bundle of His:**
special conductive tissue in the middle of the septum of the heart, or interventricular septum, that allows smooth and rapid conduction of the electrical impulse from the AV node to the ventricle.

**bundle branches:**
special conductive tissue fibers that extend from the Bundle of His and into the left and right ventricle.

**Purkinje fibers:**
conduction fibers that branch off from the bundle branches and deliver the electrical stimulus to the ventricles, causing the ventricles to contract.

From the SA node, the electrical impulses travel through the right and left atria to the **atrioventricular node**, or (**AV node**). The AV node is also composed of specialized conductive tissue and is located in the lower part of the right atrium near the junction of the atrium and ventricle, also known as the **AV junction**. The purpose of the AV node is to delay the electrical impulses coming from the SA node to allow the atria enough time to contract and deliver blood into the ventricles. In a heart that is functioning normally, the SA node regulates the heart beat. However, if the SA node fails, the AV junction serves as a back up pacemaker. The AV junction produces electrical impulses at a slower rate than the SA node, resulting in heart rates of 60 beats per minute and slower.

After leaving the AV node, the electrical impulse travels through the **bundle of His**. This is a group of specialized conductive tissue fibers that help channel the electrical current from the AV node to the lower part of the heart. The bundle of His extends from the AV node down the septum and then divides into two branches. The **right bundle branch** extends into the right ventricle, and the **left bundle branch** extends into the left ventricle. The current travels from the bundle of His, to the bundle branches, to the **Purkinje fibers**, and then out into the muscle tissue of the right and left ventricles.

To summarize electrical conduction: the SA node initiates an electrical impulse which travels throughout the atria and then to the AV node, which delays the impulse momentarily. The AV node then conducts the impulse to the bundle of His, to the bundle branches, and ultimately to the right and left ventricles. This extensive conduction system ensures that the electrical impulse is relayed in an orderly and efficient manner. If the electrical current is not coordinated, the pumping action of the heart will not be effective. The conduction system also has back up systems: the AV junction is a back up pacemaker if the SA node fails, and ventricular tissue is a back up pacemaker for the AV junction. The ventricular tissue has the slowest rate of all; it will only beat at a rate of 40 beats per minute or less.

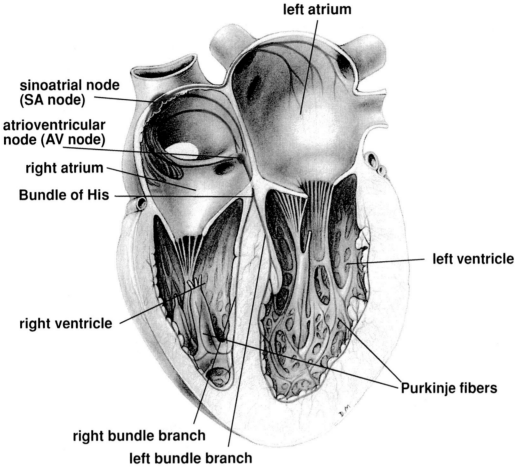

left atrium

sinoatrial node
(SA node)

atrioventricular
node (AV node)

right atrium

Bundle of His

left ventricle

right ventricle

Purkinje fibers

right bundle branch

left bundle branch

*From LifeART, Grant's Atlas1, Copyright 1999,
Lippincott Williams & Wilkins.*

The SA node initiates the electrical impulse, which travels through the right and left atria and then to the AV node. The AV node delays the electrical impulse slightly before allowing the impulse to travel to the bundle of His and then to the right and left bundle branches. The Purkinje fibers complete the electrical conduction to the heart muscle (the myocardium). This electrical stimulation causes muscle contraction.

*Figure 3-5: The Conduction System of the Heart*

# The Cardiac Cycle

The **cardiac cycle** is the series of electrical and mechanical events that comprise each heart beat. It starts at the beginning of one beat of the heart and ends with the beginning of the next beat. The synchronization (timing) and coordination (arrangement) of these electrical and mechanical events is essential for the proper functioning of the heart. As mentioned earlier in this chapter, electrical stimulation precedes mechanical contraction.

To put this very complex process simply, the cardiac cycle begins with the depolarization of the atria, which causes the atria to contract. The contraction causes the blood in the atria to empty into the ventricles. Ventricular depolarization occurs as the ventricles are filled with blood. After depolarizing, the ventricles contract. The right ventricle contracts slightly before the left ventricle and ejects blood into the pulmonary artery. When the left ventricle contracts, it ejects blood into the aorta.

**systole:**
the period of time in which the heart muscle is contracting.

The period of time when the ventricles contract is called **systole**. During this contraction, the heart is at work and producing a peak blood pressure in the aorta and arteries. Systolic blood pressure is the highest pressure produced in the arteries. This pressure is reflected in the top number of the blood pressure reading. The significance of systole is that the pressure produced must be adequate to **perfuse** the tissues and organs of the rest of the body with blood carrying necessary oxygen and nutrients.

**diastole:**
the period of time when the heart muscle is relaxed.

The period of time in which the ventricles are relaxed and not in contraction is called **diastole**. The diastolic reading (the bottom number in a blood pressure reading) represents the pressure in the arteries when the heart is at rest. Even though this resting period is brief, it is very important. The coronary arteries that feed the heart cannot fill while the heart is contracting. It is during diastole that the coronary arteries receive oxygen-rich blood to deliver to the heart.

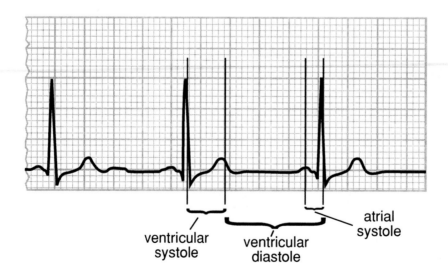

*Figure 3-6: The Cardiac Cycle. This shows the relationship between the ECG recording and the contraction/relaxation of the heart.*

Within the space of a heartbeat, an electrical current stimulates the heart. In order for the heart to contract and relax, precisely timed events must occur. These events involve the opening and closing of valves, the contraction of the atria, and then the contraction of the ventricle. The coordination and synchronization of the electrical and mechanical actions of the heart is the essence of the cardiac cycle. It is important to note that rather than being sequential in nature, some of the events in the cycle actually overlap (See Figure 3-6). For instance, contraction of the atria occurs during the end of ventricluar diastole and the beginning of ventricular depolarization. This point helps to illustrate the complexity of the cardiac cycle and emphasizes the importance of precisely-timed events to the proper functioning of the heart.

## Chapter Summary

The heart is a muscular organ composed of a series of chambers. The job of the heart is to pump blood throughout the body.

The two small chambers at the top of the heart are the atria. The large chambers in the lower part of the heart are the ventricles. The right side of the heart receives blood depleted of oxygen from the rest of the body and pumps it to the lungs. In the lungs, the blood takes up oxygen. The left side of the heart pumps the oxygenated blood to the rest of the body. The heart valves keep the blood flowing in one direction.

Electrical stimulation must precede mechanical contraction. The ECG can pick up the electrical activity of the heart. The blood pressure is a reflection of the mechanical pumping of the heart. The electrical conduction system of the heart consists of the SA node, the AV node, the bundle of His, the bundle branches, and the Purkinje fibers. The SA node is the pacemaker of the heart.

A cardiac cycle is the series of events that occur between the beginning of one heart beat and the beginning of the next heart beat. The cycle involves the coordination and synchronization of the electrical and mechanical events of the heart. Proper timing and arrangement of the events is vital to proper cardiac function.

Name_____

Date_____

# Student Enrichment Activities

**Label the heart diagram with the anatomical features listed below.**

1. right atrium
2. left atrium
3. right ventricle
4. left ventricle
5. chordae tendenae

6. tricuspid valve
7. pulmonic valve
8. mitral valve
9. aortic valve
10. papillary muscle

11. inferior vena cava
12. superior vena cava
13. pulmonary artery
14. pulmonary vein
15. intraventricular septum
16. aortic arch

*From LifeART, Super Anatomy 1, Copyright 1998, Lippincott Williams & Wilkins.*

**Describe the structures the blood flows through in order, from the right side of the heart to the left side of the heart.**

**17.** Blood returns to the heart through the _____ (1) and _____

_____ _____(2), which empty into the right _____(3). Blood flows

through the _____valve (4) and into the right _____(5); then

through the _____valve (6) and into the _____

_____(7). From there, blood is delivered to the lungs in order to pick up

oxygen and release carbon dioxide. The oxygen-rich blood then returns to the heart

through the _____ _____(8) and empties into the left

_____(9). Flowing through the _____valve (10), the blood enters

the left _____(11) and proceeds through the _____valve (12)

into the _____(13) and to the rest of the body.

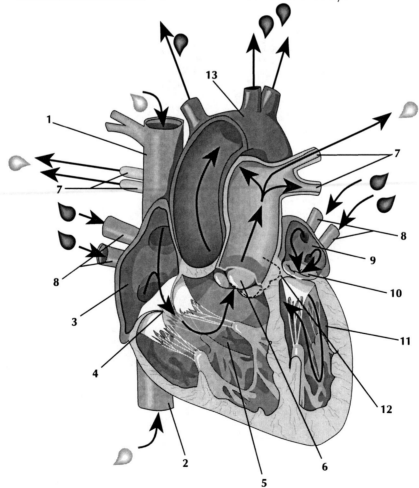

*From LifeART, Super Anatomy 1, Copyright 1998,*
*Lippincott Williams & Wilkins.*

Name_____

Date_____

**Label the heart diagram with the features of the conduction system.**

18. SA node
19. AV node
20. Bundle of His

21. Left bundle branch
22. Right bundle branch
23. Purkinje fibers

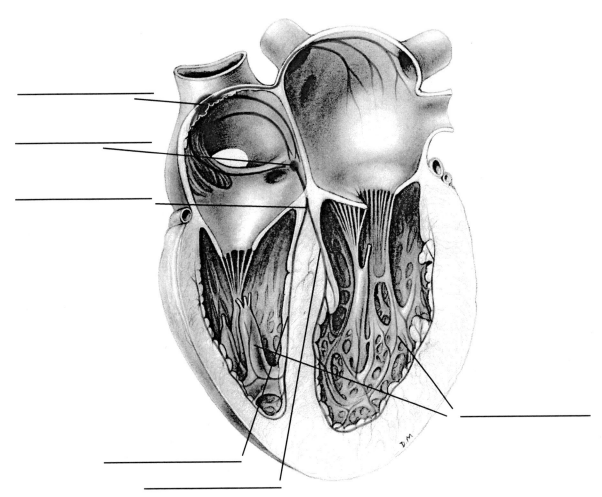

*From LifeART, Grant's Atlas 1, Copyright 1999,
Lippincott Williams & Wilkins.*

**Match the terms in Column A with the definition in Column B.**

<u>Column A</u>                                          <u>Column B</u>

24. ___ vascular

A. Special conductive tissue located in the lower right atrium.

25. ___ vena cava

B. Carries deoxygenated blood from the right side of the heart to the lungs.

26. ___ pulmonary vein

C. Special conductive tissue that extends into the right and left ventricle.

27. ___ atria

D. Receives blood from the left side of the heart to be distributed to the rest of the body.

28. ___ SA node

E. Pacemaker of the heart.

29. ___ bundle of His

F. Lower chambers or main pumping chambers.

30. ___ bundle branches

G. Relating to the lungs.

31. ___ systole

H. Conductive tissue leading from the AV node to the ventricular septum between the right and left ventricle.

32. ___ pulmonary

33. ___ pulmonary artery

I. Large vein returning deoxygenated blood to the right side of the heart.

34. ___ aorta

J. The resting phase of the heart.

35. ___ ventricles

K. Conductive tissue that transmits electrical impulses from the bundle branches to the ventricular tissue.

36. ___ AV node

L. Relating to the system of blood vessels.

37. ___ diastole

M. Carries oxygenated blood from the lungs to the left side of the heart.

38. ___ ion

N. The upper chambers.

39. ___ cardiac cycle

O. The time during which the heart is contracting or working.

40. ___ Purkinje fibers

P. The series of electrical and mechanical events that comprise each heart beat.

Q. Very small charged particle.

Name_____

Date_____

**Complete the following statements.**

41. _____ means that the heart generates its own electrical impulse spontaneously.

42. The flow of blood through the heart structures and the synchronized and coordinated function of the heart during one heartbeat is called the _____ _____.

43. The significance of the heart valves is that they ensure that blood will flow in _____ _____ and prevents blood from flowing _____ into the previous chamber or vessel.

44. The _____ _____ is a protective covering around the heart.

45. The _____ _____ is a bony structure that protects the heart, lungs, and large vessels.

46. The _____ _____ has a thick muscle and large chamber because it has to pump more blood farther than any of the other heart chambers.

47. _____ _____ must understand the anatomy and physiology of the heart in order to successfully perform their job.

48. The _____ covers the heart. The heart muscle is the _____ and the lining of the heart is the _____.

# Chapter Four
# ECG Basics: The Heartbeat as a Waveform

## *Objectives*

After completing this chapter, you should be able to
do the following:

1.  Define and correctly spell each of the key terms.

2.  Discuss how the events of polarization, depolarization,
    and repolarization relate to the ECG tracing.

3.  Describe how the electrical impulses represented by the
    ECG waveform relate to the activities of the heart chambers.

4.  Label the components of the normal sinus waveform of
    the ECG tracing.

# Key Terms

- action potential
- baseline
- depolarization
- polarization
- P wave

- PR interval
- QRS complex
- refractory period
- repolarization
- T wave

# Application of Theory

**polarization:** the period of time when the cellular membrane is in a resting state.

This chapter will describe the waveforms that compose the ECG tracing. The electrical current passing through the heart tissue is the activity that determines the ECG tracing. In the previous chapter the concepts of **polarization, depolarization**, and **repolarization** were introduced. In this chapter these actions, which take place on the cellular level, will be described in terms of waveforms that can be visualized, examined, and measured on the ECG tracing. The theory of the movement of electrolytes across a membrane (depolarization) will be applied to the ECG waveforms. The mechanical results of the electrical activities will also be discussed in terms of the ECG tracing.

**depolarization:** the period of time when ions or electrolytes are exchanged through a semi-permeable membrane and an electrical current is discharged.

**repolarization:** the period of time when electrolytes move back through the cellular membrane and a resting state is re-established.

# The Action Potential

The **action potential** is a measurement of the difference between the electrical charges on either side of the cell membrane and is an indication of the cell's capability and likelihood of discharging an electrical current. The action potential is described in terms of polarization, depolarization, and repolarization. To review, polarization is when the cell membrane is in a resting state. This means that there is a very low possibility that a current will be discharged. Depolarization is the discharge of an electrical current that occurs when ions move across a membrane. Repolarization is the repositioning of ions along the cell membrane for the purpose of restoring the resting state.

**action potential:** the difference in the electrical charge between the two sides of a cell membrane that indicates the probability an electrical current will be discharged.

These actions occur on the cellular level. The cells of the conduction system, such as the cells that compose the SA node, as well as the muscle cells of the heart have an action potential and go through the depolarization cycle. The cells of the SA node have a shorter resting phase and start to depolarize sooner and over a longer period of time than the cardiac muscle cells. This is because the SA node is the pacemaker and must initiate the electrical current.

## The Waveforms

The resting phase of the conduction cycle, or the polarized state, is visible on the ECG tracing as the **baseline**, or isoelectric line. The baseline is the straight line on the ECG tracing. It represents an absence of electrical activity. The baseline is important because the beginning of a waveform is marked by a departure (or movement away) from the baseline. The ending of a waveform is marked in terms of a return to the baseline. This is critical to understand because in order to be able to examine and measure a waveform, a clear understanding of where the waveform begins and ends is necessary. The baseline is the reference point for determining the beginning and end of a waveform.

**baseline:** the polarized state in which no perceptible electrical discharge is visible on the ECG; also called the isoelectric line.

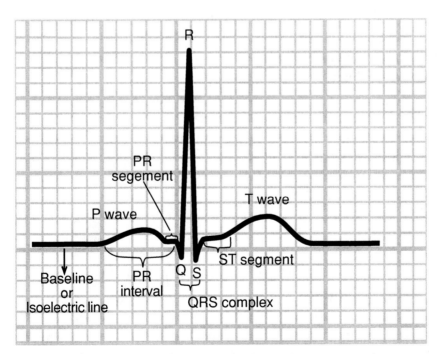

Figure 4-1: This illustration shows the baseline, the P wave, the PR interval, the QRS complex, the ST segment, and the T wave — all components of one heartbeat.

**P wave:**
the waveform on the ECG that represents atrial depolarization.

When the SA node initiates a heartbeat, it depolarizes the tissues within the SA node. This discharge sends an electrical signal to the surrounding muscle cells to depolarize also. The wave of depolarization spreads throughout the tissues of the right and left atria. The depolarization of the atria is reflected in the ECG tracing as the **P wave**. The P wave is a relatively small, rounded, and symmetrical waveform on the ECG tracing. An **interval** is the duration or length of time in which a waveform occurs and is measured in fractions of a second. A **segment** is the period of time that begins when a waveform returns to baseline and lasts until the next waveform begins. When measuring an interval, the segment following the wave form may be included in the measurement. The details of measuring waveforms will be addressed in Chapter Eight.

**QRS complex:**
a waveform on the ECG that comes after the P wave and represents ventricular depolarization.

The electrical current then goes to the AV node, where it is delayed slightly. It is then relayed to the bundle of His and the right and left bundle branches. From the bundle branches, the current moves out into the ventricular muscle and the ventricles are depolarized. Ventricular depolarization is visible on the ECG tracing as the **QRS complex**. The QRS complex is a sharp triangular waveform and is a much taller wave than the P wave. The ventricles are larger than the atria, so it takes a stronger current to depolarize them. However, the current travels faster in the ventricles, so the QRS complex takes place over a shorter period of time than the P wave. The result is that the QRS complex is a tall and narrow wave when compared to the P wave. The **PR interval** is the duration of the P wave and is measured in fractions of a second. It is measured from the beginning of the P wave to the beginning of the R wave.

**PR interval:**
the time period from the onset of the P wave to the beginning of the R wave.

**T wave:**
the waveform on the ECG that represents ventricular repolarization and occurs after the QRS.

After depolarization, the ventricles repolarize; the resting state is restored. Ventricular repolarization is reflected in the **T wave**, which occurs after the QRS complex. The T wave has a rounded gentle curve, is taller than the P wave, and has a longer duration than the QRS complex. Only the repolarization of the ventricles is visible on the ECG tracing. Repolarization of the atria, which occurs after the P wave, occurs at the same time as the QRS complex and is buried in that wave.

**refractory period:**
the time during repolarization when the cardiac cell cannot respond to another electrical impulse.

During the repolarization stage a **refractory period** occurs. The refractory period is the time during repolarization when the cardiac cell would not be able to respond to another electrical impulse. The refractory period occurs right after the QRS complex and during most of the T wave. It is not a waveform, but describes the condition of the cardiac muscle during repolarization. An electrical impulse cannot be conducted in tissue that is repolarizing. In the latter part of repolarization (the last part of the T wave), most of the tissue is recovered, and an impulse may be conducted at that time.

After the T wave, a U wave may be visible. The U wave is a small rounded wave that is not always distinct on the ECG tracing. It is thought that the U wave may represent repolarization of the Purkinje fibers. It is not measured and not significant unless it is prominent or larger than expected, because then it may indicate a disease condition. After the T wave (or U wave if it is present) the tracing returns to baseline, reflecting a brief resting period for the myocardium. Then the cycle begins again.

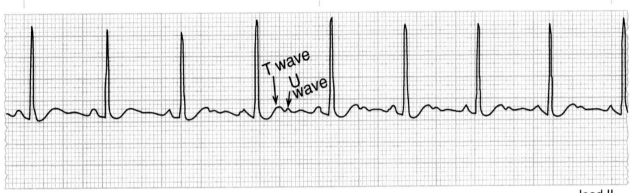

lead II

*Figure 4-2: The U wave is not always present on the ECG tracing. A relatively small U wave is a normal variation. Large and prominent U waves may indicate electrolyte imbalance or medication toxicity.*

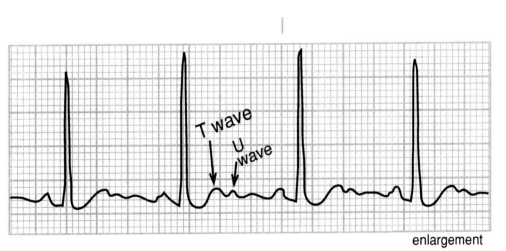

enlargement

*Figure 4-3: (Enlargement of Figure 4-2.) If a U wave is present, it will occur just after the T wave.*

# The Cardiac Cycle

When looking at the ECG tracing, it is important to remember that it represents the electrical function of the heart and that there is a corresponding mechanical action. The electrical function is an electrical impulse that initiates the contraction, which results in the pumping of the heart. One P wave and QRS complex represent one heartbeat. One heartbeat generates a pressure which creates a pulse that is felt in distal parts of the body such as the wrist. The constant pumping of the heart sustains the forward movement of blood to other parts of the body. The pressure created by this pumping is the blood pressure. None of this could happen without the electrical activity represented on the ECG tracing. It is equally important to remember that the ECG tracing is not the same as blood pressure and pulse, but is part of the cycle and the coordination of the electrical and physical actions of the heart.

To summarize: the atria depolarize, creating a P wave on the tracing; the impulse travels to the AV node, bundle of His, bundle branches, and the Purkinje fibers; the ventricles depolarize, then contract. The ventricular contraction ejects blood into the aorta, causing a blood pressure and pulse to be produced. This is the normal cardiac cycle . Disease may cause a disruption in these events, adversely affecting heart function, blood pressure, and pulse. The ECG can be used to obtain information about the disease process and heart function.

# ECG Tracing

This chapter has discussed the activities in the heart that are represented by the ECG, as well as the result of these activities. So how do the ECG waveforms become a tracing on paper? How is this tracing examined and used to form a diagnosis? The detailed procedure of obtaining an ECG will be discussed in the next chapter. The purpose of this section is to summarize the process, equipment, and end result.

Initially, a patient is connected to an ECG machine using special attachments called **sensors**, or electrodes, which are attached to the chest at specific locations near the heart. Cable wires connect these sensors to the electrocardiograph, which can detect the electrical activity in the heart. The electrocardiograph is also a recording device; it translates the electrical signals into a tracing on paper. The paper tracing then can be studied, and the waveforms can be measured.

The paper used for the tracing is a grid or graph type of paper. The grid is created by numerous horizontal and vertical lines that create small and large squares. The small squares are made with light lines. Every five small squares make up a large square that is marked by dark lines. The **horizontal** lines (those going across the page) measure time. The **vertical** lines (those going up and down) measure voltage or electrical current. Each small square represents 0.04 seconds. Each large square represents 0.2 seconds. These time intervals will be important to know when examining the heart rhythms and measuring the waveforms.

## Chapter Summary

The electrical conduction system of the heart is critical to the proper functioning of the heart. The electrical activities of the heart occur at the cellular level and involve the movements of ions across a semipermeable membrane. This movement of ions causes an electrical current, which results in the mechanical contraction of the heart muscle.

The ECG reflects the electrical activity of the heart. The ECG consists of waveforms that represent the polarization, depolarization, and repolarization of the atria and ventricles of the heart. The waveforms are labeled the P wave, which is atrial depolarization; the QRS complex, which is ventricular depolarization; the T wave, which is ventricular repolarization; the U wave, which is thought to be repolarization of the Purkinje fibers; and the baseline, which represents the polarized state. A segment is the part of the ECG tracing that is between two waves. An interval is the length of a wave with a segment.

The ECG waveforms are recorded by an electrocardiograph on special paper that is calibrated to measure the duration of the waves created by the electrical current. This ECG recording, called a tracing, can then be examined by a nurse or physician. The information obtained from an ECG tracing can be used by a physician to help form a diagnosis of the patient's condition.

Name_____

Date_____

# Student Enrichment Activities

**Match the terms in Column A with the appropriate definition in Column B.**

## Column A

1. ___ polarization

2. ___ depolarization

3. ___ repolarization

4. ___ P wave

5. ___ QRS complex

6. ___ T wave

7. ___ baseline

8. ___ action potential

9. ___ refractory period

10. ___ ECG graph paper

11. ___ PR interval

12. ___ ST segment

## Column B

A. The difference between the electrical charges on either side of the cell membrane, which represents the likelihood for the movement and subsequent discharge of an electrical current.

B. The waveform on the ECG that represents atrial depolarization.

C. The period of time in which the cell membrane and electrolytes are in a resting state.

D. The time during repolarization when the ventricle cannot respond to an electrical stimulus.

E. The waveform that represents ventricular repolarization.

F. The state in which ions move across a semipermeable membrane and discharge an electrical current.

G. The polarized state in which little or no perceptible electrical discharge is visible on the ECG.

H. Waveforms on the ECG that represent ventricular depolarization.

I. The period of time in which the electrolytes move back toward the resting state.

J. Horizontal lines represent time and vertical lines represent voltage.

K. The period of time from the beginning of the P wave to the beginning of the R wave.

L. The return to baseline from the end of the S wave to the beginning of the T wave.

**Label the ECG waveforms on the tracing below.**

13.

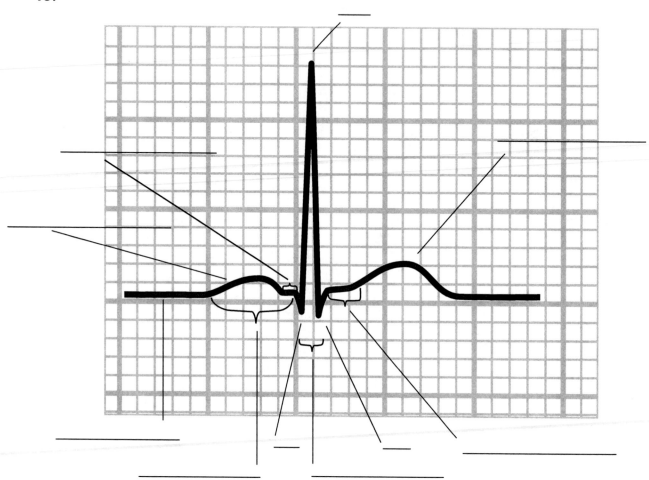

Name_____

Date_____

**Complete the following statements.**

14. _____ stimulation precedes the _____ events in the heart.

15. The mechanical pumping of the heart creates the _____ _____ and the _____.

16. _____ and _____ are the means by which the ECG machine is attached to a person.

17. The ECG machine translates _____ _____ into a waveform that can be analyzed.

18. Atrial _____ is represented on the ECG tracing as the P wave.

19. The _____ _____ is a rapid, sharply-formed wave that represents ventricular depolarization.

20. The T wave represents ventricular _____ and is a rounded waveform.

21. The _____ _____ represents the likelihood that an electrical current will be discharged.

# Chapter Five
# The 12-Lead ECG

## *Objectives*

After completing this chapter, you should be able to
do the following:

1.  Define and correctly spell each of the key terms.

2.  Describe what a "lead" is and identify the 12 leads used in
    a standard ECG.

3.  Describe the equipment used when obtaining an ECG.

4.  Demonstrate how to prepare a patient's skin for an ECG and
    explain why proper preparation is important.

5.  List the steps to be followed when taking an ECG.

6.  List potential causes of artifacts on the ECG recording.

7.  Perform an ECG.

# Key Terms

- artifact
- cable
- calibration
- galvanometer
- graph paper
- ground lead

- isoelectric line
- lead
- pericarditis
- sensor
- stylus
- ventricular hypertrophy

# Introduction

The value of accurately performing the steps of the ECG procedure cannot be overemphasized. If the procedure is done incorrectly, the quality of the ECG tracing will be compromised and an accurate diagnosis may not be made. Enlisting the patient's cooperation is an essential part of the process of obtaining a high-quality ECG. It is important to remember that human interaction is just as vital as the handling of equipment.

# Indications for an ECG

The ECG contains a tremendous amount of valuable information for the healthcare team. Trained healthcare professionals, such as physicians and nurses, can interpret or "read" the ECG. This means that deviations in the ECG can be assigned a particular meaning and a diagnosis can be made. A certain medical treatment may be prescribed based on the results and subsequent interpretation of the ECG. Therefore, it is crucial that the ECG be accurate so that proper treatment will be prescribed.

**pericarditis:**
inflammation of
the pericardial
sac covering
the heart.

**ventricular
hypertrophy:**
enlargement of
the ventricle.

An ECG is helpful in diagnosing or confirming ischemia (poor blood flow to the heart muscle), MI (severe decreased blood flow that results in myocardial cell death), **pericarditis** (inflammation of the pericardial sac surrounding the heart), or **ventricular hypertrophy** (enlargement of the ventricle). An ECG also is helpful in detecting electrolyte imbalances and in performing rhythm analysis.

A physician may order an ECG if the patient is experiencing chest pain, tightness or pressure in the chest, light-headedness, or shortness of breath. The ECG is then used to determine if these symptoms are related to functions of the heart. The ECG may provide one part of the puzzle and other tests may be ordered to fill in the missing pieces so that a proper diagnosis can be made.

An ECG may also be ordered as part of a routine physical examination in a clinic, physician's office, or in a hospital setting. The ECG is then used to compare with future ECGs to see if there is any deviation or change. As a patient's condition changes over time, it is often helpful to have an ECG from his or her past for comparison purposes.

Critical care nurses are trained in **12-Lead ECG** interpretation. They can detect changes and critical developments that show up on the ECG. They are then responsible for communicating this information to the physician. This timely interpretation allows the patient to be treated quickly for abnormalities rather than having to wait for the physician to make his or her rounds.

## Preparing the Patient

It is important to remember that the patient may be apprehensive because he or she is in pain or frightened about the outcome of his or her present health problems. In addition, the patient may not be acquainted with the hospital or clinic procedures, which can add to his or her distress. It is the responsibility of all healthcare team members to keep the patient informed about the environment and procedure he or she will be experiencing.

To prepare a patient for an ECG, you must first verify that the physician has ordered an ECG for him or her. To do this you may need to look at the patient's chart or talk directly with the physician or nurse. Then, verify that you have the correct patient by checking his or her name band or directly asking the patient to state his or her name.

As an ECG technician you are responsible for explaining the environment, equipment, and procedure to the patient. Explain that you will be connecting the patient to the ECG machine in order to obtain information about his or her heart function. It needs to be made clear that this information will help in the formation of an accurate diagnosis and the development of the best plan of care for the patient.

**sensor:**
a disc or tab made of plastic that has a metal component as well as a layer or well of gel or conducting substance, and which is placed on a patient's skin in order to pick up electrical activity from the heart where it is transmitted through cables to the ECG machine to be processed. Also called an electrode.

Reassure the patient that the procedure is painless and will only take about 15 minutes. Explain that **sensors** (electrodes) will be attached to his or her arms, legs, and chest. These sensors are then attached to lead cables, which are connected to the ECG machine. Electrical information is transmitted from the surface of the skin to the sensors and through the cables to the electrocardiograph to be processed. The machine then records the information from the heart onto graph paper. After providing this explanation, ask the patient if he or she has any questions or concerns. If necessary, reassure the patient that there is no risk in performing this test.

Once you have explained the procedure to the patient, instruct him or her to take off the clothing on the upper part of the body and give him or her a gown to wear. Because the skin on the patient's legs must be easily exposed, the patient also will need to take off tight pants or pantyhose. Have the patient lie flat on his or her back with arms at the sides and legs straight. Remind the patient to lie very still so that the recording will be accurate. Talking and breathing can affect the quality of the ECG, so remind the patient not to talk or take deep breaths; he or she should breathe normally and be very still.

It is important to be respectful and sensitive to the patient's needs and concerns. Allow the patient privacy when removing his or her clothing. If the patient needs help in removing clothing, use a gentle touch and be sensitive. It may be necessary for a male patient with a very hairy chest to have small areas of the chest shaved where the sensors need to be applied. Ask him for permission to do this if it is deemed necessary. Gently shave the areas using a dry razor.

Areas on the skin surface where sensors are to be placed must be free of natural oils, lotions, and perspiration. Cleansing the skin will ensure proper conduction of electrical impulses from the skin surface to the electrode. Clean the area with alcohol or soap and water. Use dry gauze or a cloth towel to dry the area. The roughness of the dry gauze helps to remove dead skin and other substances that will get in the way of conduction.

# The Electrocardiograph

The electrocardiograph is the machine used to obtain the electrocardiogram (ECG). Remember that the ECG is not an indicator of blood pressure or the actual mechanical contraction of the heart, but of the electrical events in the heart. It is a measure of the electrical activity that stimulates the contraction of the heart. The electrocardiograph has sensors, amplifiers, and various features that are designed to gather this electrical information and translate it into readable data in the form of a tracing. The electrocardiograph was first developed in the early 1900s. William Einthoven, a Dutch physiologist designed the original machine. This was a breakthrough in medical technology for which Einthoven won the Nobel Prize in 1924. The triangle shown in Figure 5-9B is called the Einthoven triangle.

In order to pick up the heart's electrical signals, the sensors are placed on the patient's body at strategic locations. The locations of the sensors give information about different locations of the heart. There are 10 different locations for the sensors in a standard ECG, which result in 12 different **views** of the heart. The 12 views are also called "12 **leads**." The 12-Lead ECG is the standard ECG that is done most of the time. The 12 different views and the placement of the sensors will be explained and described later in the chapter.

**lead:**
a configuration of positive and negative sensors, or electrodes, on the body surface that picks up the electrical information from the heart. The different sensor configurations offer different "views" of the heart.

The sensor is of vital importance because it is the first link between the patient and the machine. Older sensors were made of metal and were clumsy to use. They stayed in place with a suction device or rubber strap. They had to be used with gel between the metal and the patient's skin to facilitate conduction. Now the sensors are small plastic tabs that are usually sandwiched together with a very thin metal layer and a thin gel layer. The gel layer also acts as an adhesive which helps it stick to the patient's skin. The new sensors are easier to apply and take less time to place than the older sensors. They are also more comfortable for the patient. The tabs are less than an inch square and are very thin. Newer sensors have a rounded, nonadhesive tip that is attached to the ECG lead **cables**. The cables have clamps at the end that grab the tip of the sensor tabs. If the patient has to have serial ECGs (several ECGs done in a short amount of time) the plastic tabs can be left in place so that they can be used the next time an ECG is needed. Leaving the tabs in place increases the efficiency and accuracy of the serial ECG. Even a small variation in the placement of a sensor will make the ECG waveform look different. So if the tabs are left in place, future ECGs will be more accurate and meaningful. If changes are detected, it will indicate actual changes in the heart and not a change in sensor location.

**cable:**
one or more insulated wires that connect sensors to an electrocardiograph.

Once placed, the sensor picks up electrical activity from the skin surface. This electrical activity is then transmitted from the sensor along the cable to the electrocardiograph machine. The cable is a metal wire that is insulated by a thick plastic covering. The electrical current travels along the metal wiring.

When the electrical signal reaches the electrocardiograph machine, the signal is amplified and processed. The electrical activity that is transmitted from the heart to the skin is only a few millivolts; so, in order to be diagnostically useful, it must be amplified about twenty billion times. After amplification, the electrical impulse travels to the **galvanometer**, which transforms the electrical impulse into mechanical motion. The mechanical action directs the movement of the **stylus**, which forms a tracing on the **graph paper**. The resulting lines and curves created on the graph paper are called waveforms. These are the waves that are studied by the physician and nurse. This tracing is usually made by a chemical coating on the graph paper that reacts to heat in the tip of the stylus.

The ECG machine requires a power source in order to function. Many ECGs are designed to be used with an internal battery. The machine is plugged into a wall socket only when not in use in order to charge the battery. This is a helpful feature because it creates less electrical interference during a test than an ECG machine that is plugged into an outside power source. When the machine is plugged in and the battery is charging, a small light may appear on the control panel. A power switch may be located on the control panel or on the side or back of the machine. But machine models may differ. The technician will have to be instructed in the proper use of the specific model being used at the facility where he or she is employed.

Many different kinds of electrocardiographs are in use today. They differ in physical appearance and design. This is a general introduction to the features common to most ECG machines. There have been many recent advances in medical technology that have affected the design of ECG machines. New machines are capable of recording three or more channels (leads) at one time. Older machines were only capable of recording one channel at a time. Thus, obtaining an ECG was more time-consuming and interpreting the tracings was more difficult. The multichannel recorders are able to get more information in less time. Some machines have a screen where the ECG waveforms can be viewed before they are printed. This allows adjustments to be made before the tracing is printed. If the tracing is not clear, then the sensors may need to be reapplied.

**galvanometer:** a device in the ECG machine which detects electrical currents from a patient and converts it into mechanical energy, which is then recorded onto graph paper.

**stylus:** the needle of the ECG machine that forms a tracing on the graph paper.

**graph paper:** paper on which the ECG is recorded that is preprinted with horizontal lines representing time and vertical lines representing voltage.

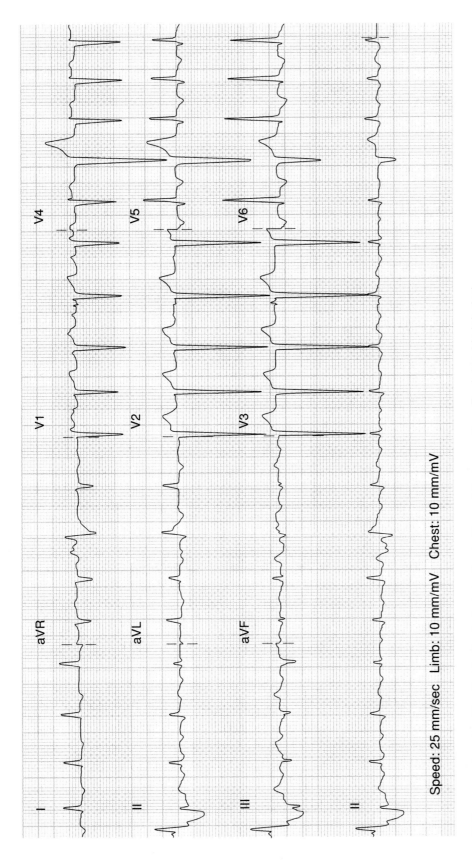

Speed: 25 mm/sec   Limb: 10 mm/mV   Chest: 10 mm/mV

Notice speed and calibration indicated along the bottom of the recording. Each lead is labeled.

*Figure 5-1: A 12-Lead HP Multichannel ECG Recording*

Prominent features on electrocardiographs commonly include the following:

The *record* switch initiates the recording of the ECG waveforms onto the graph paper. The paper is fed through the area of the machine where it comes in contact with the stylus, and the recording is made.

**calibration:**
the process of setting a machine to a standardized scale so the results will be comparable and tests can be compared.

The *standardization* control is important to ensure accuracy and to apply a universal **calibration**. This control creates a standardization mark on the ECG paper that reflects machine calibration. By international agreement, this mark must be 10mm high and 2mm wide (see Figure 5-4). If the mark does not meet this specification, then the machine must be recalibrated. Calibration enables machines made by different manufacturers to use the same units of measure and allows comparisons to be made between ECGs that have been run on different machines. This calibration standardizes the measurement of voltage and the precision of the waveform, and ensures that the amplitude of the waveforms on the ECG accurately represents the electrical activity of the patient's heart. This will be discussed in more detail later in the chapter. Newer machines calibrate automatically.

The *stylus heat control* setting determines the lightness or darkness of the markings. When the heated stylus touches the specially coated graph paper, a chemical reaction occurs. This reaction is what produces the markings. A hotter stylus makes a thicker, darker line and a cooler stylus makes a lighter, thinner line. Again, machines by various manufacturers may operate slightly differently. On some machines, this feature may have a different name or be programmed for automatic adjustments.

**artifact:**
additional electrical activity on an ECG tracing as a result of muscle movement, alternating current (AC), or disruption of the cable, rather than the electrical activity of the heart.

The *frequency control* or **filter** acts to filter out extra electrical activity from the environment that may interfere with the recording. Extra waves on the recording that do not represent heart activity are called **artifacts**. Having the filter feature activated will help to diminish artifacts from the recording. Artifacts reduce the quality of a recording, so it is important to recognize and eliminate them.

The *lead selector* designates which view of the heart will be recorded. Most machines can be run on either manual or automatic. When the machine is set on automatic, the leads to be recorded are preprogrammed and will automatically record the 12 leads needed for the standard ECG. Multichannel recorders usually can record three leads at a time. If additional leads are needed, then adjustments can be made to include extra leads. On older machines that do not have an automatic setting, the leads are recorded one at a time and the machine may need to be put on *stand by* while the lead selector is adjusted.

On older machines the *marker* button may need to be pressed in order to indicate which lead is being recorded. These machines use a code to mark the various leads being recorded. Otherwise, the technician must manually mark the leads (See Figure 5-2 for codes). Most newer machines will label the leads automatically.

| Limb Leads | Code | Chest Leads | Code |
|------------|------|-------------|------|
| I | _ | $V_1$ | _ _ |
| II | _ _ | $V_2$ | _ _ _ |
| III | _ _ _ | $V_3$ | _ _ _ _ |
| aVR | _ _ | $V_4$ | _ _ _ _ _ |
| aVL | _ _ _ | $V_5$ | _ _ _ _ _ _ |
| aVF | _ _ _ _ | $V_6$ | _ _ _ _ _ _ _ |

*Figure 5-2: Older machines (not multichannel recorders) that record only one lead at a time may use a code to identify each lead recorded.*

When using an older ECG model, the technician has to be patient and persistent in order to obtain a high quality recording. Recording only one lead at a time is very time consuming, uses more graph paper, and requires the cutting and mounting of the leads in the appropriate order.

The newer computerized models or multichannel recorders are easier to use because they record three leads simultaneously and arrange all 12 leads on an 8 X 10 piece of graph paper. The leads are already arranged and marked in the proper order. These tracings are easier to handle and analyze.

The multichannel recorders have other convenient features as well. For example, they usually have a keyboard so that the patient's name, age, and medications can be listed and entered on the ECG paper. This information appears in the heading on the same page as the ECG. Multichannel recorders also have a memory that can store ECGs for a period of time. If the printed copy is lost, the stored ECG can be reprinted.

Computerized machines are able to measure waveforms, note abnormalities, and give a preliminary diagnosis from the recording. The diagnosis given by the machine is only a guide and must be confirmed by a physician or nurse—the healthcare professional may disagree with the computer diagnosis. The physician's interpretation is the diagnosis that is entered into the patient record. Even so, these machines are valuable and assist the healthcare professionals obtaining accurate data about the heart.

As we have seen, major advances in computer science and medical technology have influenced the art of obtaining a 12-Lead ECG. But there are limitations too. This is still a machine that is only as good as the technician who is putting it to use. Proper technique is still needed to assure an accurate recording. The most important part of this technique is proper placement of the sensors. Procedures for operating the machines may vary, but sensor placement for the chest leads does not. Sensor placement will be described in detail later in the chapter.

## The ECG Recording

Like all graph paper, ECG graph paper has preprinted horizontal and vertical lines. The horizontal lines measure time and the vertical lines measure electrical voltage. The squares created by the lines measure 1 millimeter (mm) in length. Every fifth line is marked with a heavy line, creating a pattern of squares that are composed of lighter and darker lines. This assists in the reading of the ECG. The smaller 1mm squares are outlined by lighter lines, and the larger 5mm squares are outlined by darker lines. The smaller squares along the horizontal axis represent increments of 0.04 seconds or 4/100ths of a second. Thus, five small horizontal squares, or one heavy square equals 0.2 seconds or 1/10th of a second. This information will be important in a later chapter when analyzing the waveforms.

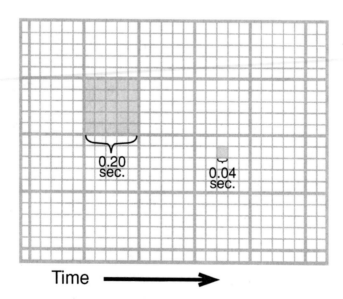

Times travels along the horizontal axis from left to right.
The large box represents 0.2 seconds and the small box
represents 0.04 seconds.

*Figure 5-3: Time and ECG Paper*

A knob or button on the ECG machine is used to regulate the speed at which the paper is fed through the machine and past the stylus. When the indicator is set at speed 25, then the machine will move the graph paper at a rate of 25mm per second or 25 small boxes per second; the same as 5 large boxes per second. This is the usual rate for the standard ECG and produces the characteristic waveform that is easily recognizable.

When the indicator is set at speed 50, then the paper will go at a rate of 50mm or 50 small boxes per second; that's twice as fast as it would go if it was set at speed 25. The use of speed 50 creates a waveform that is stretched out and elongated from what it would look like at speed 25. If speed 50 is used, it must be clearly indicated on the recording or the resulting waveform will be misinterpreted because the waveform recorded at speed 50 will make the heart rate appear slower than the recording done at speed 25. This faster speed may be useful in examining complex, fast heart rhythms or when one wave may be hiding in another. The stretching out of the waveform allows for a more accurate analysis of certain complex heart rhythms. It is not used in the standard ECG, but may be used in rhythm analysis. Remember, if speed 50 is not clearly indicated on the ECG paper, an inaccurate diagnosis could be made, resulting in an inappropriate intervention or treatment for the patient.

The vertical lines on the graph paper are used to indicate voltage. This measures the strength of the electrical current that is being produced by the heart. Ten small boxes or two large boxes on the vertical axis equals 1cm (centimeter). By international agreement, 1cm is equal to 1 millivolt. This universalizes the 12-Lead ECG and standardizes measurements and interpretation. Whenever an instrument is used to measure a particular item, the instrument must be **calibrated** in order to ensure accuracy of the measurement. When something is calibrated it means that a standard measurement is being used as a reference. Older machines require manual calibration. Newer machines calibrate automatically at the beginning of each new lead. A calibration marking is a squared-off wave that indicates that the machine has been reset to the reference measurement.

If the voltage coming from the patient is so low that the resulting wave is difficult to read, then the machine can be calibrated to a different scale. The *sensitivity control* adjusts this scale and increases the output of the amplifier. This process is also referred to as *gain*. Usually the sensitivity control is set at 1 or 1 millivolt. However, it could be set at 2, which would double the output of the amplifier, resulting in a taller waveform. If a patient's ECG demonstrated a recording in which the waveforms were too tall and were "squared-off" or which ran off the page, then the gain could be adjusted to 1/2. This would allow the whole waveform to be printed on the tracing.

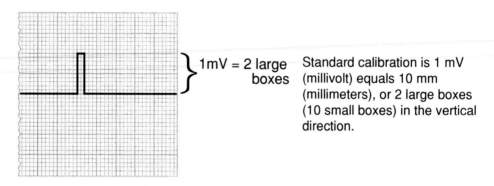

1mV = 2 large boxes    Standard calibration is 1 mV (millivolt) equals 10 mm (millimeters), or 2 large boxes (10 small boxes) in the vertical direction.

*Figure 5-4: Voltage and ECG Paper*

The *position control* is important because it determines where the baseline of the ECG will be located on the graph paper. Remember, the baseline is the horizontal line which the stylus makes when there is little or no electrical activity that can be picked up by the ECG machine. It may also be called the **isoelectric line**, meaning that the electrical state is balanced and there is no movement of current.

**isoelectric line:** the baseline; a straight line on the ECG recording that represents an absence of electrical activity.

In order to ensure that the waveform is easy to read, the waveform should be centered appropriately on the graph paper. The position control can adjust the placement of the waveform so that it is centered. This helps the technician to prepare an accurate and complete recording. If the position control is not adjusted properly, the waveform may run over the edge of the paper at either the top or bottom.

# Lead Placement and Description

The standard ECG is called a 12-Lead ECG because it uses 12 leads to obtain information about the heart. This means 12 views, or angles, of the heart are used to reflect information about different areas of the heart. The proper placement of the sensors is vital to obtaining an accurate ECG recording.

Anatomical landmarks are parts of the body or skeleton that can be easily seen or palpated (felt with the hands). Detailed information about specific anatomical landmarks is required in order to assure precise placement of the sensors.

## Anatomical Landmarks

Remember that the heart lies in the center of the chest with the **apex**, or bottom, of the heart tilted toward the left. The main landmarks include the **clavicle**, the **sternum**, the **ribs**, the **intercostal spaces**, and the **axilla**. The heart lies within the borders of these structures.

A **clavicle** is a collarbone. The right clavicle and left clavicle are located on the top of the right and left side of the torso, respectively. Each clavicle is a curved bone that extends from the base of the neck to the shoulder. The clavicles protrude slightly and are easily palpated (felt) on the right and left sides of the chest. Now, imagine a vertical line on the left side of the chest that separates the left clavicle into two equal portions. Extend this line down the chest **parallel** to the arm. This line should come close to the inside of the left nipple. This is called the **midclavicular line** and is a major reference point used when examining the heart and listening to heart sounds with a **stethoscope**. It is a critical reference point used to correctly place ECG leads.

The **sternum** is the breastbone and is the firm, flat surface in the center of the chest. The sternum is divided into three parts: the manubrium, the main body of the sternum (gladiolus), and the xiphoid process. The manubrium is the top part of the sternum. The clavicles attach to the manubrium. A groove at the top of the manubrium is called the presternal notch, or the jugular notch. The middle portion of the sternum is commonly called the main body of the sternum. Attached to the bottom of the sternum is a small bone called the **xiphoid process**. References to the sternum will usually be in terms of the **sternal border** (the edge of the sternum along the outline of the bone), and will specify the "right" or "left" sternal border. Another important reference is the Angle of Louis, which is the raised ridge where the manubrium and the sternum come together.

The **ribs** form a bony cage that protects the heart and lungs. The first rib is located just beneath the clavicle. Immediately below the clavicle is the first **intercostal space**. The intercostal spaces consist of cartilage and muscle which hold the ribs together. When running the fingers down the chest, one can feel the alternating firm ridges of the ribs with the indented, softer valleys of the intercostal spaces.

The intercostals are used as landmarks to locate proper placement of the ECG sensors. Each intercostal space shares the number of the rib directly above it. (eg, the first intercostal follows the first rib.) The first intercostal is just below the first rib and the clavicle. Remember, the first rib is just behind the clavicle and cannot be palpated, but the clavicle can be easily located. Next is the second rib, then the second intercostal, and so on down the chest.

It is sometimes difficult to locate and count the ribs and the intercostal spaces. On patients who are very thin it will be easy to detect and count the ribs and the intercostal spaces. For patients who are obese, have deformities of the chest, or have very large breasts, it will be difficult to determine the exact landmarks. Determining where these landmarks are is an essential skill for an ECG technician—one that will improve as the technician acquires more experience.

Another landmark is the **axilla** (the area under the arm). The midaxillary line is an imaginary line down the middle of the axilla that runs parallel to the arm when it is held straight against the side. The anterior axillary line is the imaginary line that descends from the anterior axillary fold. This line forms the border of the front of the chest and the axillary region. The posterior axillary line is the imaginary line that descends from the posterior axillary fold. It forms the border between the back of the torso and the axillary region. Each of the axillary lines are imaginary lines that run parallel to the arm and down the entire trunk of the body.

## A. Front (Anterior) View

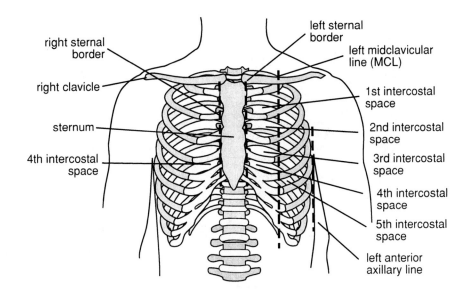

## B. Side (Lateral) View

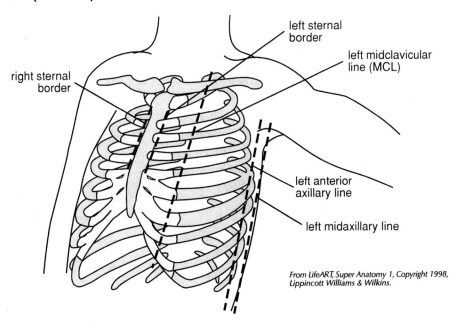

From LifeART, Super Anatomy 1, Copyright 1998,
Lippincott Williams & Wilkins.

*Figure 5-5: Anatomical Landmarks for Chest Leads*

**A. Front (Anterior) View**

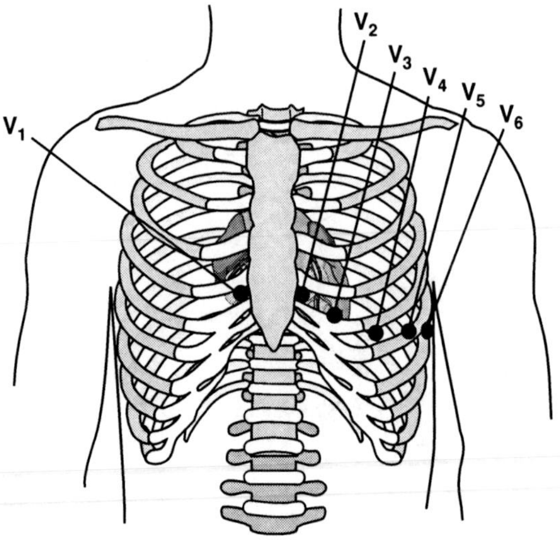

$V_1$ - Right Sternal Border in the
        4th Intercostal Space

$V_2$ - Left Sternal Border in the
        4th Intercostal Space

$V_3$ - Halfway Between $V_2$ and $V_4$

$V_4$ - Midclavicular Line in the
        5th Intercostal Space

$V_5$ - Anterior Axillary Line at the
        Same Level as $V_4$

$V_6$ - Midaxillary Line at the
        Same Level as $V_4$

**B. Side (Lateral) View**

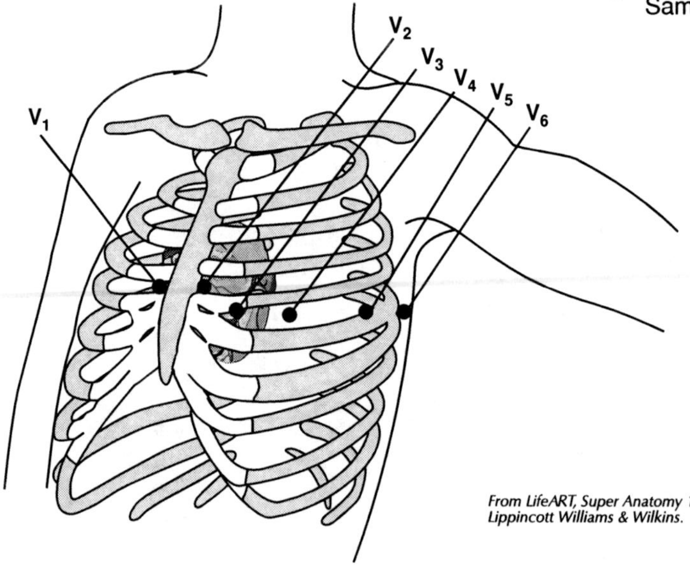

*From LifeART, Super Anatomy 1, Copyright 1998,
Lippincott Williams & Wilkins.*

*Figure 5-6: Chest Leads*

Important landmarks are also found on the arms and legs. Flat, fleshy areas are preferred, so the arm sensors are usually placed either on the inner aspect of each forearm or the lateral surface of the upper arm. The inner aspect (medial aspect) of both the legs at the lower calves is the usual placement area for the legs.

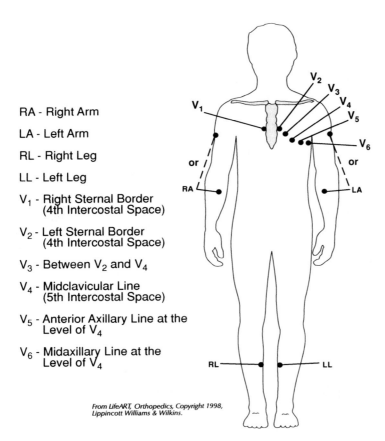

RA - Right Arm

LA - Left Arm

RL - Right Leg

LL - Left Leg

V$_1$ - Right Sternal Border
      (4th Intercostal Space)

V$_2$ - Left Sternal Border
      (4th Intercostal Space)

V$_3$ - Between V$_2$ and V$_4$

V$_4$ - Midclavicular Line
      (5th Intercostal Space)

V$_5$ - Anterior Axillary Line at the
      Level of V$_4$

V$_6$ - Midaxillary Line at the
      Level of V$_4$

*From LifeART, Orthopedics, Copyright 1998,
Lippincott Williams & Wilkins.*

*Figure 5-7: Lead Placement*

Every patient's torso looks a little different. There is a wide range of normal. Differences must be noticed. For instance, variations that deform the spine, such as scoliosis and kyphosis, also change the shape of the chest and make it difficult to find landmarks. As mentioned previously, obesity and large breasts can also obscure landmarks. The whole purpose of using landmarks is to assure consistent and accurate sensor placement so that every patient will have an ECG that accurately represents what is going on in his or her heart. This consistency allows for valid comparisons of recent and past ECGs. By following the sensor placement guidelines and correctly identifying the landmarks, the ECG will remain a valid tool that can be used to interpret disease states and identify deviations from the norm—even when a patient is very large or very small, or otherwise has an unusual chest shape.

Sometimes the tabs or sensors can be left on the patient who is undergoing a serial ECG for a day or two, until the series of ECGs is completed. But sometimes this is not practical, or the sensors become displaced by patient movement. Therefore, the proper use of anatomical landmarks also will ensure that a patient undergoing a serial ECG will have sensors placed in the same place, even when taken by different technicians.

## Anatomical Function and ECG Recordings

When recording or reading an ECG, it is useful to visualize the heart in its three dimensional space. It is also useful to remember its anatomy and physiology. The heart is located along the lower half of the sternum, and is tilted back and toward the left.

The right side of the heart is much smaller than the left side. This fact follows a rule of thumb that states, "function dictates form." The function of the right side of the heart is to pump blood to the lungs. This is a relatively short distance through a relatively small number of blood vessels. The function of the left side of the heart is to pump blood to the rest of the body through a relatively large number of blood vessels. This is why the left side of the heart is larger than the right side. The standard ECG is designed primarily to reflect the function of the left side of the heart. Most of the leads reflect the activity of the left side of the heart.

Each of the 12 leads is designed to reflect electrical activity from a specific area of heart muscle. The various leads register the electrical activity in the different walls of the heart. The surface of the heart is divided into five sections. The **anterior wall**, **anteroseptal wall**, **lateral wall**, **inferior wall**, and the **posterior wall**.

The **anterior wall** is the front part of the left ventricle and comprises the main portion of the left side of the heart. It lies directly beneath the left side of the chest. Therefore, the ECG sensors that are placed over the left chest directly reflect the anterior portion of the heart. This means that when the ECG sensors are placed on the left chest, the primary electrical current that is detected is from the anterior wall. However, a fainter, secondary current can also be detected from the posterior wall. This secondary current is referred to as an "indirect reflection." The positioning of sensors is described in terms of anatomical landmarks. Thus, the anatomical landmark for the anterior wall of the heart is the left chest, ribs 2 through 5.

The **anteroseptal wall** or region is the area of the heart that extends from the anterior wall to the septum. Remember that the septum is the wall that separates the right and left ventricles. The anatomical landmark for the anteroseptal wall is along the left sternal border.

The **lateral wall** or region is located on the side of the heart that is facing the left arm or left axilla. Remember, the axillary lines are the anatomical landmarks used for lead placement. The anterior axillary line is an imaginary line down the front of the chest that starts at the front fold of the underarm, or axilla; the midaxillary line is a line down the side from the mid portion of the underarm.

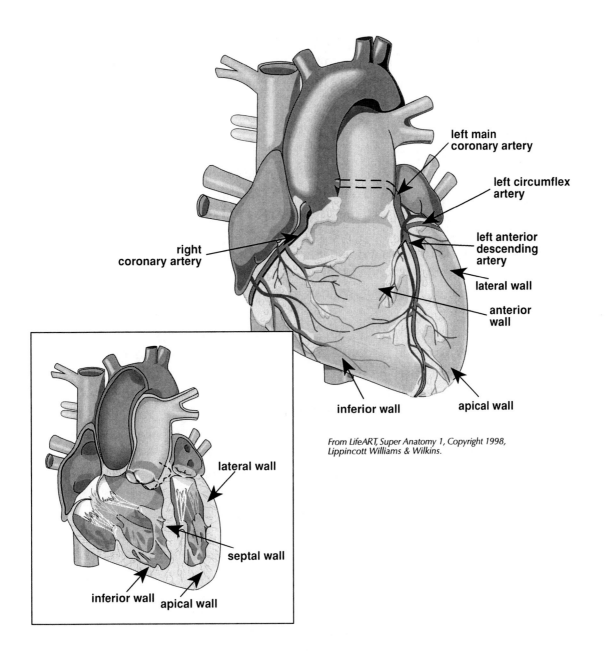

left main
coronary artery

left circumflex
artery

left anterior
descending
artery

lateral wall

anterior
wall

right
coronary artery

inferior wall

apical wall

*From LifeART, Super Anatomy 1, Copyright 1998,
Lippincott Williams & Wilkins.*

lateral wall

septal wall

inferior wall    apical wall

*Figure 5-8: Coronary Arteries and Walls of the Heart with Inset Showing a
Crossection of the Septal Walls*

Because the heart is tilted, the bottom portion of the heart that lies over the
**diaphragm** is referred to as the **inferior wall** of the heart. The wall includes
inferior portions of the left and right ventricle. If more information about the right
ventricle is needed, then extra leads in addition to the standard 12 leads can be
ordered and placed on the right side of the chest. The placement of the right
chest sensors mirror the placement of the left side sensors (the exact placement
of the sensors will be discussed later.)

The **posterior wall** is the region opposite the anterior wall, facing the spine. Sensors can be placed on the left side of the back to record direct electrical activity of the posterior (back) of the left ventricle, although this is not the usual placement for a 12-Lead ECG.

## The Leads

As stated earlier, leads are different angles, vantage points, or perspectives from which to view the heart. Each lead looks at different walls of the heart and provides information about the damage or condition of the heart muscle in that area. Leads are created by placing the sensors at specific locations on the body. From these different locations, the sensors sense the flow of electricity and determine whether the electrical current is going toward the sensor or away from it. This electrical activity determines how the waveforms look.

Some leads are **bipolar**, and others are **unipolar**. Sensor placement does not change from lead to lead – only sensor usage changes. The electrocardiograph is programmed to use the properly placed sensors to create these unipolar or bipolar leads. Bipolar leads have both a negative and a positive sensor. The positive sensor in any lead is the "looking" sensor; it is the vantage point from which the heart is being examined or viewed. The negative sensor has the opposite polarity of the positive sensor. These two sensors set up the angle for viewing the heart. In the bipolar leads the ECG measures the difference of the electrical energy between two points, the positive and the negative sensor. This is then translated into a waveform. If the current is going toward the positive sensor, then the wave will be positive (it will rise from the baseline, or isoelectric line). If the current is going away from the positive sensor, then the wave will be negative (it will descend from the baseline).

Unipolar leads consist of only a positive sensor. The negative sensor exists at an imaginary point created by the positions of the remaining leads. The positive sensors are placed on the body and the electrocardiograph calculates the theoretical placement of the negative sensor by internally processing the electrical impulse of the heart. The result is similar to the results of a bipolar lead: the current traveling toward the sensor will be recorded as a positive waveform, and the current traveling away from the sensor will be recorded as a negative waveform.

## The Standard Limb Leads

The limb leads refer to the leads that are obtained from placing the sensors on the arms and legs. The limb leads are **Lead I**, **Lead II**, and **Lead III**. The limb leads are the bipolar leads, meaning that it is necessary to have two sensors physically placed on the patient in order to measure the electrical activity. Each lead utilizes two of the three active sensors. They record activity on the frontal plane of the heart. One sensor is placed on each limb; one on each arm and leg. The right leg (RL) sensor is the "**ground lead**," meaning it is not used to determine electrical activity, but rather it is used as a reference point. In the bipolar limb leads, the galvanometer measures the difference in electrical potential between two sensors.

**ground lead:** a lead that is not used to determine electrical activity, but rather as a reference point.

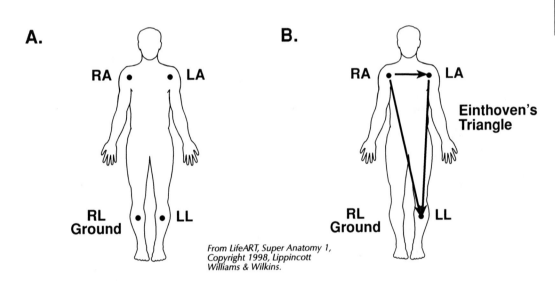

From LifeART, Super Anatomy 1, Copyright 1998, Lippincott Williams & Wilkins.

**A.** Four limb sensors or electrodes are used to record cardiac voltage. They are: Right Arm (RA); Left Arm (LA); Left Leg (LL); and Right Leg (RL).

**B.** Remember, the Right Leg electrode is the "ground" or reference sensor. It is a reference point and does not provide actual cardiac information. The three active sensors are used to record three leads, or views, of the heart: Lead I, Lead II, and Lead III. These three leads are the standard limb leads. Each of these leads are bipolar, using two of the three active sensors. Lead I, Lead II, and Lead III form Einthoven's triangle.

*Figure 5-9: Limb Sensors (B shows Einthoven's Triangle.)*

In Lead I, the sensor on the right arm (RA) is negative and the left arm (LA) sensor is positive. This lead detects the flow of electrical current through the heart on the plane between the right and left arm. The positive sensor, which is on the left arm, is the view point of this lead. If you look at the heart from the left arm, then you will see the lateral portion of the left ventricle. Therefore, this lead reflects the condition of the lateral wall of the heart.

In Lead II, the right arm sensor is negative and the left leg (LL) sensor is positive. This lead detects the flow of electrical current through the heart on the plane between the right arm and the left leg. The positive sensor is looking up at the heart from the viewpoint of the left leg. This lead reflects information about the inferior wall of the heart.

In Lead III, the left arm sensor is negative and the left leg is positive. Again the positive sensor is looking up at the heart from the leg. This lead detects the flow of electrical current through the heart on the plane between the left arm and the left leg. This lead also reflects information about the inferior wall of the heart. Lead II and Lead III are referred to as the inferior leads (the leads that reflect the condition of the inferior wall). If an infarction was noted in these leads by an elevation of the ST segment, then the diagnosis would be an inferior wall myocardial infarction. The ECG helps to pinpoint the location of the damage to the heart.

As you can see, in the bipolar leads, sometimes a sensor is needed as a positive sensor and sometimes as a negative sensor, depending on the lead that is being recorded. When selecting the lead settings on the 12-lead ECG, the machine will adjust the sensor from positive to negative automatically.

## A. Lead I

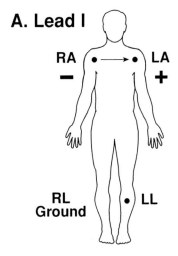

Lead I records the electrical current through the heart, from the right arm to the left arm.

RA Sensor is negative.

LA Sensor is positive.

The heart is viewed from the positive electrode, or LA, which views the *lateral wall* of the heart.

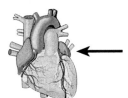

## B. Lead II

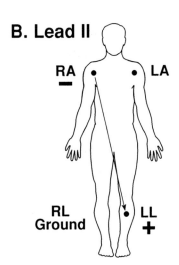

Lead II records the electrical current downward through the heart's long axis, from the right arm to the left leg.

RA Sensor is negative.

LL Sensor is positive.

The heart is viewed from the positive electrode, or LL, which views the *inferior wall* of the heart.

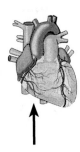

## C. Lead III

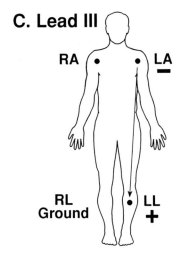

Lead III records the electrical current from the left arm to the left leg.

LA Sensor is negative.

LL Sensor is positive.

The heart is viewed from the positive electrode, or LL, which views the *inferior wall* of the heart from another angle.

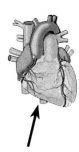

*Body outline and heart illustrarion from LifeART, Super Anatomy 1, Copyright 1998, Lippincott Williams & Wilkins.*

*Figure 5-10: Standard Limb Leads*

## The Augmented Leads

Augmented leads are unipolar leads meaning that only one positive sensor is used to obtain the electrical information and that they measure the electrical current from one point. Remember, the positive sensor is the "looking" sensor. The negative reference consists of an imaginary point configured by the remaining limb leads. The electrocardiograph calculates this reference point which is centered around the heart. The configuration of the augmented leads results in an amplitude increase of 50% over the standard limb leads. This enhances the resulting waveform. The abbreviation for **augmented voltage** is "aV."

The augmented leads make use of an exploring positive sensor. The two sensors opposite the exploring sensor are transformed by the electrocardiograph into a negative reference point. Then the electrocardiograph measures the difference between the electrical potential directly beneath the exploring sensor and an imaginary line drawn from the positive sensor in use to a point midway between two remaining sensors. Just as the standard limb leads do, the augmented leads look at the heart from the frontal plane.

The augmented lead of the right arm is abbreviated "aVR." The exploring positive sensor is the right arm. The view of the heart is from the right shoulder and into the center of the heart cavity and reflects activity from the top of the heart. So, aVR is the recording of the electrical current through the heart along the axis from the midpoint between the left arm and left leg to the positive pole of the right arm.

The abbreviation, "aVL," refers to the augmented lead of the left arm. The exploring positive sensor is the left arm. The view of the heart is from the left shoulder and reflects the information from the lateral or high lateral wall of the heart. Thus, aVL records the electrical current through the heart along the axis from the midpoint between the right arm and left leg to the positive pole of the left arm.

The augmented lead of the left foot is abbreviated "aVF." The exploring positive sensor is the left foot. The view of the heart is from the left foot up to the heart and reflects information from the inferior wall of the heart. Thus, aVF is a recording of the electrical current through the heart along the axis from the midpoint between the right arm and left arm to the positive pole of the left leg.

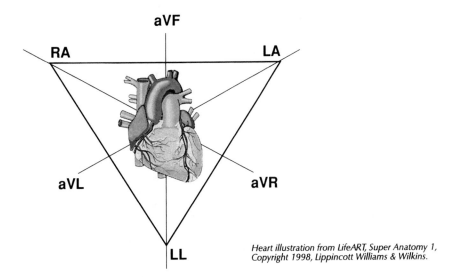

Heart illustration from LifeART, Super Anatomy 1, Copyright 1998, Lippincott Williams & Wilkins.

The augmented leads make use of all three active sensors to record three additional views of the heart: aVR, aVL, and aVF. Each of the augmented leads are unipolar, measuring voltage from one point. The negative reference point is determined by the computer within the electrocardiograph.

*Figure 5-11: The Views of the Augmented Leads*

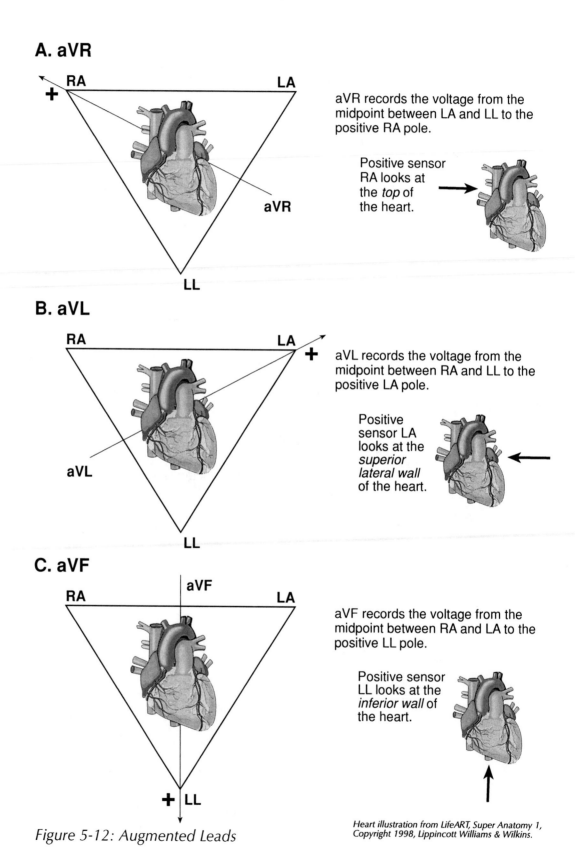

## A. aVR

aVR records the voltage from the midpoint between LA and LL to the positive RA pole.

Positive sensor RA looks at the *top* of the heart.

## B. aVL

aVL records the voltage from the midpoint between RA and LL to the positive LA pole.

Positive sensor LA looks at the *superior lateral wall* of the heart.

## C. aVF

aVF records the voltage from the midpoint between RA and LA to the positive LL pole.

Positive sensor LL looks at the *inferior wall* of the heart.

*Figure 5-12: Augmented Leads*

*Heart illustration from LifeART, Super Anatomy 1, Copyright 1998, Lippincott Williams & Wilkins.*

## Precordial leads

The **precordial leads** are the chest leads. They are also unipolar leads. Their positions are positive and the negative reference is an imaginary point located toward the posterior or back, created by the limb leads. The precordial leads look at the heart on a horizontal plane, from a front to back perspective. The limb leads looked at the heart from a side to side and an up to down perspective.

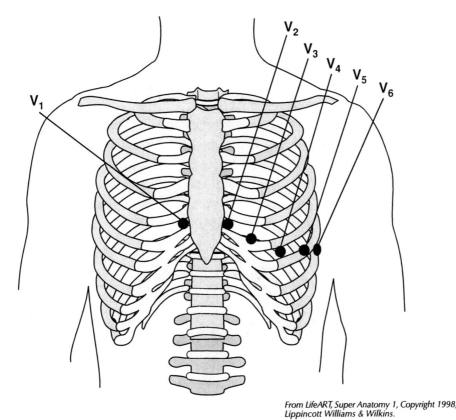

*From LifeART, Super Anatomy 1, Copyright 1998, Lippincott Williams & Wilkins.*

$V_1$
$V_2$
$V_3$ } These leads look at the interventricular septum and anterior wall.

$V_4$ } This lead looks at the anterior wall.

$V_5$
$V_6$ } These leads look at the apical and low lateral walls.

*Figure 5-13: Precordial Leads*

There are six chest leads: $V_1$, $V_2$, $V_3$, $V_4$, $V_5$, and $V_6$. Lead $V_1$ is located at the right sternal border over the 4th intercostal space. It looks at the anteroseptal portion of the heart, toward the interventricular septum. $V_2$ is located at the left sternal border over the 4th intercostal space. Lead $V_3$ is located between $V_2$ and $V_4$. Lead $V_4$ is located on the midclavicular line, over the 5th intercostal space. Leads $V_2$ and $V_3$, like $V_1$, look at the anteroseptal portion of the heart. $V_4$ looks at the anterior wall of the heart. Lead $V_5$ is located on the left anterior axillary line, at the level of the 5th intercostal space. Lead $V_6$ is located on the left midaxillary line, at the level of the 5th intercostal space. Leads $V_5$ and $V_6$ both look at the apical and low lateral walls of the heart.

An optional lead is $V_4R$ meaning the $V_4$ lead is to be obtained from the right side of the chest. This lead may be requested if a right ventricular infarction is suspected. The sensor would be placed at the 5th intercostal space on the midclavicular line on the right side of the chest. Similarly, a $V_7$, $V_8$, and $V_9$ can be ordered if a posterior infarction is suspected. Sensors for these leads are placed by locating the left 5th intercostal space and following this level around the chest to the back. $V_7$ is at the posterior axillary line; $V_9$ is at the midpoint of the left back; and $V_8$ is between $V_7$ and $V_9$.

# Procedure for Obtaining a 12-Lead ECG

A 12-Lead ECG is begun by assisting the patient to a comfortable position on his or her back (the supine position). The patient should be informed about the need for the ECG and that his or her cooperation is both needed and appreciated.

As discussed earlier, there are many different kinds of electrocardiographs; from single channel recorders to state-of-the-art multichannel recorders. The following procedure is intended to be a general outline that will apply to most ECG machines.

# Obtaining a 12-Lead ECG

**Materials needed:**

✓ an electrocardiograph with patient cables and loaded with ECG graph paper
✓ electrodes or sensors
✓ gauze pads
✓ skin cleanser
✓ a disposable razor

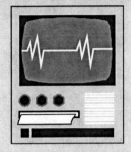

1. Procedural Step: Wash your hands before touching the patient or any equipment.
   Reason: Pathogens (germs) can be passed along to a patient any time there is contact with a healthcare worker. As healthcare workers, we strive to help the patient improve their physical ailments and not acquire new ones.

2. Procedural Step: Identify the patient.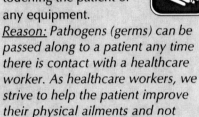
   Reason: You must always make sure that you have the correct patient.

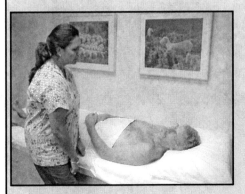

3. Procedural Step: Explain the procedure and the equipment to the patient.

Reason: If a patient understands the procedure, as well as its purpose and usefulness, then the patient will be more cooperative and less frightened.

4. Procedural Step: Ask the male patient to remove clothing so that the chest is completely bare and the arms and the lower part of the legs are bare and accessible. A gown that opens in the front should be worn by the female patient. With the use of a drape, a skillful technician can preserve the patient's modesty while properly placing the sensors.
   Reason: In order to find the anatomical landmarks, place the sensors correctly, and obtain an accurate ECG, clothing must be removed from the body parts that require the placement of sensors.

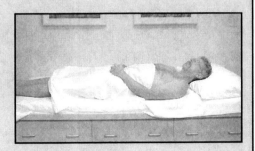

# Obtaining a 12-Lead ECG (Cont.)

5.  Procedural Step: Make sure that the ECG machine has a charged battery or is plugged in and that the power switch is on.
    Reason: All ECG machines require a power source to run. Some have a battery that is used when taking the ECG and then charged when not in use. Others need to be plugged into the wall in order to run.

6.  Procedural Step: Make sure that the patient's skin is clean and dry. If a male patient has an unusually hairy chest, then ask him if you may shave his chest. Shave only small 1-inch square areas where the sensors are to be placed. Briskly rub the areas where the sensors are to be placed with a terry cloth towel or gauze pads to remove dead skin and to increase circulation.

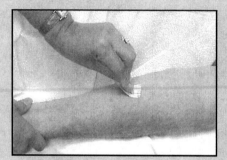

    Reason: It may be necessary to wash and dry the skin in areas where the sensors are to be placed. This is necessary if the patient is perspiring and the skin is damp or if the patient has heavy lotion on the skin. Alcohol-saturated pads will remove oils and lotions. Skin is a relatively poor conductor of electricity, so removing dead skin cells and increasing circulation are necessary to improve conduction.

7.  Procedural Step: Place one sensor, or electrode, on each limb. The inner aspect of the calves is generally used for the RL and LL sensors. For the RA and LA sensors, some manufacturers recommend the inner surface of the forearm. Other manufacturers recommend the lateral surface of the upper arm instead of the forearm to reduce the risk of artifacts due to muscle movement. If using an older machine, then gel will have to be applied to the skin, the metal sensor placed over the gel, and then a rubber strap attached to hold the sensor in place. If a newer system is in use, then a disposable sensor is used. The sensor is a plastic tab that has a thin layer of a metallic substance on the back side, which is then covered with a thin coating of the adhesive gel. The gel side is placed against the patient's skin and should easily stick there.

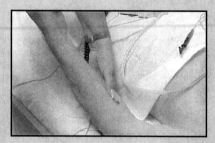

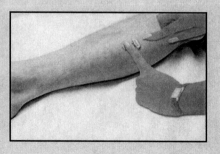

# Obtaining a 12-Lead ECG  (Cont.)

*Reason:* *Placing the sensors away from bony prominences decreases artifacts called somatic tremors.*

8. <u>Procedural Step:</u> Find the anatomical landmarks on the chest for the V leads and apply sensors, or electrodes. Locate the sternum and the sternal border. On the sternum, locate the ridge of the Angle of Louis, adjacent to the second rib. Follow the ridge to the second rib. Just below that is the second intercostal space, then count down to the fourth intercostal space along the right sternal border. This is lead $V_1$.

9. <u>Procedural Step:</u> Repeat on the left side: count down to the fourth intercostal space along the left sternal border. This is $V_2$.

10. <u>Procedural Step:</u> Locate the mid point on the left clavicle. Follow the midclavicular line down to the 5th intercostal space. This is $V_4$.

11. <u>Procedural Step:</u> Locate the mid point between $V_2$ and $V_4$, this is $V_3$.

12. <u>Procedural Step:</u> $V_5$ is located at the level of the 5th intercostal on the anterior axillary line.

13. <u>Procedural Step:</u> Follow the line at the level of the 5th intercostal space around to the side of the chest. Locate the midaxillary line by identifying the mid point of the underarm space, and follow that down to the level of the 5th

intercostal space. This is $V_6$.
**Note:** If an older machine is used, a floating disc sensor may need to be used for the chest leads. If that is the case, the gel will need to placed in each of the six V lead positions and the sensor moved to each location after each lead is recorded. If a multichannel recorder is being used, then it will be necessary to place all of the sensors on the chest before recording. In this case it is easier to use the pre-gelled sensor tabs.

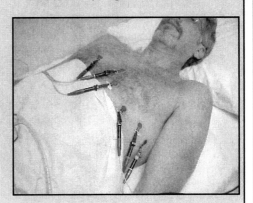

*Reason:* *Operation of ECG machines may vary according to the manufacturer and the age of the machine. New machines are less cumbersome to operate. Older machines make use of the floating disc sensor, which is placed at each of the V lead locations sequentially. This means that the sensor is placed at $V_1$ and that lead is recorded. Then the sensor is placed at $V_2$ and that lead is recorded. This is repeated until all V leads are recorded.*

# Obtaining a 12-Lead ECG  (Cont.)

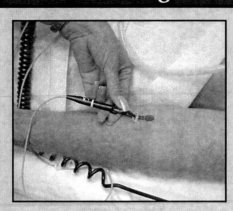

14. Procedural Step: Connect the appropriate lead cable to each sensor. Make sure that the leads are attached to the correct sensor. They are usually color-coded or have initials on each lead. Avoid having the leads and cables tangled or looped.
*Reason: If the cables are hooked up to the wrong sensor, then an inaccurate recording will be made. Tangled or looped cables can cause interference and inaccurate recording.*

15. Procedural Step: Enter the patient's name or identification number, the day's date, and the time into the machine, if it allows you that option. If the machine does not have this capability, you will have to manually write that patient's information on the recording paper when the ECG is complete.
*Reason: It is vital to identify any test or documentation related to patient care to prevent mix up or loss of information.*

16. Procedural Step: Make sure the sensitivity switch is turned to 1 (1cm equals 1 millivolt).
*Reason: This is the setting that gives the best tracing for most patients. The sensitivity can be adjusted if necessary.*

17. Procedural Step: Newer machines automatically calibrate themselves at the beginning of each lead; but, if you are using an older machine you must press the STD (standardization) button at the beginning of each lead. The standardization mark is a squared-off waveform that is exactly 10mm high (10 boxes) and 2mm wide.

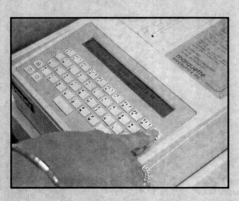

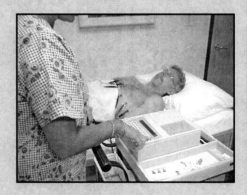

# Obtaining a 12-Lead ECG  (Cont.)

*Reason: This ensures that the measurements are consistent with international standards and have minimal distortion.*

18.  Procedural Step: Record the ECG. Make sure to have the machine turned so that you can see the patient while recording the ECG. This allows you to view any changes in the patient's condition while you are recording the tracing. Activate the filter button on the machine if necessary to help eliminate artifacts caused by interference from other electrical devices being used in the facility. However, while using the filter may be necessary, it may blur the tracing. Therefore, it is important to read the manufacturer's recommendations and to consult your facility's guidelines regarding the use of the filter. With the filter button either on or off, as appropriate, press **Record** or **Run**.
If using a single channel recorder, check the position of the stylus and reposition it if the recording is not centered. Run two or three standardization marks, then run several complexes in Lead I and insert a standardization mark between the complexes or waveforms. Record the rest of the leads in the same way. Each lead should have a standardization marking and there should be 2 or three standardization marks at the end of the 12 leads. Newer single channel recorders will automatically insert standardization marks and select and mark the leads. In older machines you may need to select the various leads and push the button that marks or labels the leads. If using a single (floating) disc V sensor, run a 6 second strip in $V_1$ and then press Standby. Move the sensor to $V_2$. Record and repeat for all V leads.

If the machine is a multichannel recorder, it will automatically label the leads and switch from one group of three leads to the next.
*Reason: With automatic settings this is very easy. The leads to be recorded are programmed into the memory of the ECG machine. For example, on multichannel recorders, usually Lead I, II, and III are recorded simultaneously, then the aVR, aVL, and aVF leads are recorded simultaneously. Then, $V_{1-3}$ are recorded, followed by $V_{4-6}$. At the bottom of the sheet a continuous tracing, usually of Lead II is recorded. (See Figure 5-1) So, by pushing just one button, 12 leads are recorded and a rhythm strip is produced. Sometimes the multichannel recorder will have a display screen that gives a preview of the 12 leads so that adjustments can be made if the waveform isn't clear. If a display screen isn't present, then an indicator may be present on the machine or on the cables that can alert the technician if the signal isn't clear. An **X** may appear for each lead in the indicator prompt if the signal isn't coming through, or a signal bar may appear if the machine is receiving a clear signal.*

---

## Obtaining a 12-Lead ECG  (Cont.)

19. <u>Procedural Step:</u> Disconnect the patient and help him or her to clean the gel off the skin if necessary. Leave the patient in a comfortable position on the bed or exam table.
    <u>*Reason:*</u> *Allowing the patient to get comfortable will help to relieve any anxiety the patient may feel about having the test.*

20. <u>Procedural Step:</u> Recheck documentation. Make sure that the name of the patient, the time, the date, the patient's age, the physician, and any medications have been noted and correctly entered into the ECG database.
    <u>*Reason:*</u> *It is essential that the name of the patient is correct and that the other information is available to the physician interpreting the results of the ECG.*

---

## Artifacts

Artifacts have been mentioned several times throughout this chapter. An accurate, high quality, and easy-to-read ECG is the ECG technician's goal. Therefore, he or she must recognize and be able to minimize or eliminate artifacts.

If there is not sufficient gel under the sensors, or if pregelled disposable sensors have dried out, then conduction from the skin's surface to the electrode and cable will be impaired and an artifact will be visible on the recording. Artifacts are lines on the tracing that obscure the waveform. Locating the defective lead is done by a process of elimination. If the artifact is noted in Leads I and II, then it may be supposed that the sensor on the right arm is causing the problem, since Leads I and II share the RA electrode. If Leads I and III show an artifact, then the sensor they share, LA, may be the culprit. If Leads II and III display an artifact, then the sensor they share, LL, may be at fault.

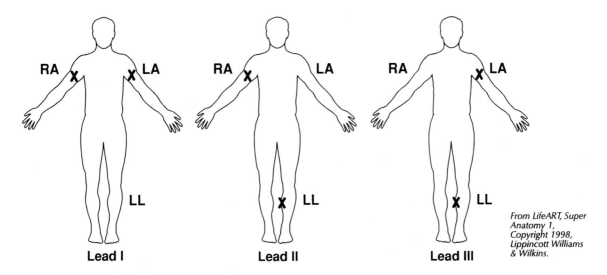

From LifeART, Super Anatomy 1, Copyright 1998, Lippincott Williams & Wilkins.

If an artifact appears in the ECG tracing, note which leads contain the artifact. Then check the sensor that is shared by those leads.

*Figure 5-14: Troubleshooting Artifacts*

A somatic tremor is caused by patient movement or tremors. To minimize this type of artifact, talk with the patient to make him or her more relaxed. Reinforce the purpose of the test and explain to the patient that accurate results require him or her to lie very still and to take only shallow breaths. Taking a deep breath during the recording will cause interference with the waveforms. Ensure that the table or bed is comfortable for the patient and that it is flat. Make sure the patient is warm enough. If the patient has a condition that causes trembling, it may be useful to have him or her put his or her hands under his or her buttocks as he or she lies on the bed.

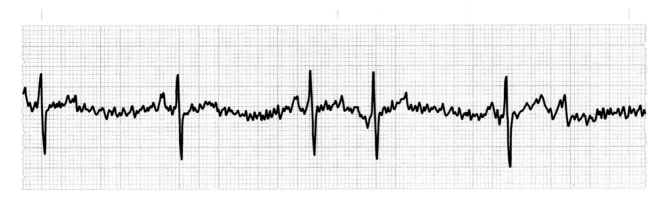

*Figure 5-15: Poor Connections. The baseline is obscured by extra squiggly lines that do not represent the activity of the heart. This can be caused by poor electrode contact with the skin or defective cables.*

A wandering baseline is usually the result of a loose limb lead connection. It may also be the result of an inadequate amount of gel on the sensor. In order to correct this, check the limb leads and secure the connections of the cables and sensors. Use adequate amounts of gel if using the older method. If using the newer method (pre-gelled sensors), check the sensors for dryness and replace them as appropriate. Be aware of the date on the package and use the older supplies as you receive new stock. A wandering baseline can also be caused by the patient sighing or taking a deep breath.

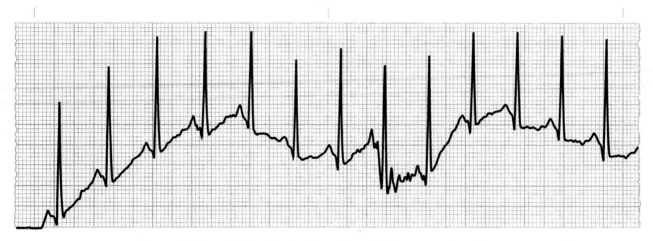

*Figure 5-16: A Wandering Baseline. This type of artifact is caused by patient movement, such as deep breathing.*

Lotions or creams on the patient's body can cause interference with the transmittal of the electrical signal. Either the signal will not be transmitted at all, or it will look erratic with a lot of extra lines in the waveform that obscure the heart signals. If you observe this, cleanse the skin with a skin cleanser or alcohol and then dry the area by briskly rubbing with a clean towel or gauze to remove the interfering substance and the dead skin. Reapply the gel and sensors.

An exaggerated, erratic waveform can be caused by a broken or loose cable. Check all cables to make sure that they are all intact and securely fitted.

Sixty cycle, or AC interference, can be caused by other electrical equipment in the area. To prevent this, make sure the ECG machine is properly grounded and has a three-pronged plug if it does not operate on a battery. If the machine operates on a battery, always run the test using battery power. Keep the machine plugged in when it is not in use to ensure that the battery is adequately charged for patient testing. Keep all cables flat, straight, and along body lines. Keep other appliances and power cords away from the patient. If possible, unplug any unnecessary electrical equipment in the area. NEVER UNPLUG ANYTHING WITHOUT FIRST CHECKING WITH THE NURSE IN CHARGE.

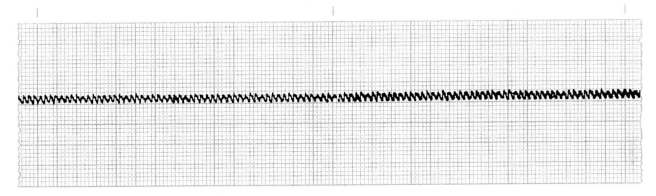

*Figure 5-17: Electrical interference from electric sources outside or within the ECG machine or monitor causes the thick zigzag baseline of a 60-cycle artifact.*

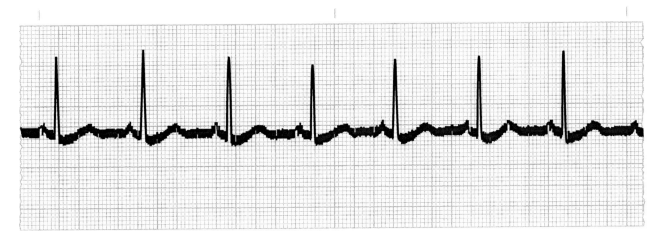

*Figure 5-18: 60-Cycle Artifact Obscuring the Baseline AND Waveforms on the ECG Tracing*

# Chapter Summary

The ECG technician's main tool, the electrocardiograph, has become easier to use over the years. These machines now have many more programmable features than they once did. As a result, the process of taking an ECG has become much more efficient than it used to be. For example, multichannel recording not only speeds the process of taking an ECG, it also provides a document that is easier for the healthcare workers to read and study.

Lead placement is based on the theory that electrical signals are transmitted from the heart to the surface of the skin and picked up by sensors placed on the skin near the heart. It is essential for the ECG technician to have an understanding of the anatomy of the heart and its position in the chest in order to understand the location of the lead placement. In addition to accurate placement of the leads, patient relaxation and cooperation is crucial to obtaining an accurate ECG.

Recognizing and troubleshooting artifacts on the ECG is also important to the quality of the ECG recording.

Name_____

Date_____

# Student Enrichment Activities

**Complete the following statements.**

1. The ECG recording represents _____ activity of the heart, whereas blood pressure and pulse represent the _____ activity.

2. Symptoms such as _____, _____, and _____ would be reasons that a physician might order an ECG.

3. The ECG can provide information about the heart and reveal conditions such as _____, _____, and _____.

4. The straight line across the ECG graph paper that means the absence of perceptible electrical activity is called the _____ or _____line.

5. A(n) _____ deflection is caused by electrical energy moving toward the positive sensor.

6. A(n) _____ deflection is caused by electrical energy moving away from the positive sensor.

7. ECG stands for _____ . It is the recording of _____ signals from the heart.

8. A multichannel recorder records _____ or more _____ simultaneously.

9. A 12-Lead ECG has three types of leads _____, _____, and _____.

10. The _____ leads view the heart on a horizontal plane, from front to back.

11. The _____ and _____ leads view the heart from an up and down, left to right perspective.

**Circle the correct answer.**

12. The electrocardiograph:
    A. measures electrical activity of the heart.
    B. has an amplifier that increases the electrical signal coming from the heart 20,000,000,000 times.
    C. prints the ECG waveform on specially coated graph paper.
    D. All of the above.

13. The standard 12-Lead ECG:
    A. is the only tool the cardiologist needs to diagnose heart disease.
    B. was invented by Einstein.
    C. provides 12 different views of the heart.
    D. is not helpful in diagnosing coronary artery disease.

Name_____

Date_____


**Match each lead in Column A with its proper anatomical landmark in Column B.**

<u>Column A</u>                                                    <u>Column B</u>

14. ___ ground

15. ___ lead I

16. ___ lead II

17. ___ lead III

18. ___ aVR

19. ___ aVL

20. ___ aVF

21. ___ V$_1$

22. ___ V$_2$

23. ___ V$_3$

24. ___ V$_4$

25. ___ V$_5$

26. ___ V$_6$

**A.** fourth intercostal space, left sternal border

**B.** negative sensor on the right arm, positive on the left leg

**C.** exploring sensor left arm, positive

**D.** fourth intercostal space, right sternal border

**E.** negative sensor right arm, positive left arm

**F.** exploring sensor right arm, positive

**G.** fifth intercostal space, midclavicular line

**H.** exploring sensor foot, positive

**I.** negative sensor left arm, positive left leg

**J.** right leg

**K.** fifth intercostal space, midaxillary line

**L.** fifth intercostal near the anterior axillary line

**M.** between V$_2$ and V$_4$

Match each lead in Column A with the view of the heart that it provides in Column B. Hint: more than one may apply.

<u>Column A</u>

<u>Column B</u>

27. ___ lead I

**A.** inferior wall

28. ___ lead II

**B.** high lateral wall

29. ___ lead III

**C.** lateral wall

30. ___ aVL

**D.** anteroseptal wall

31. ___ aVF

**E.** anterior wall

32. ___ $V_1$

33. ___ $V_2$

34. ___ $V_3$

35. ___ $V_4$

36. ___ $V_5$

37. ___ $V_6$

**Complete the following exercise.**

38. Perform a standard 12-Lead ECG on a fellow student.

Name_____

Date_____

**Analyze the following rhythms.**

**39.** • Rate _____        Acceptable Quality Recording?

 • Regularity _____            Yes        No

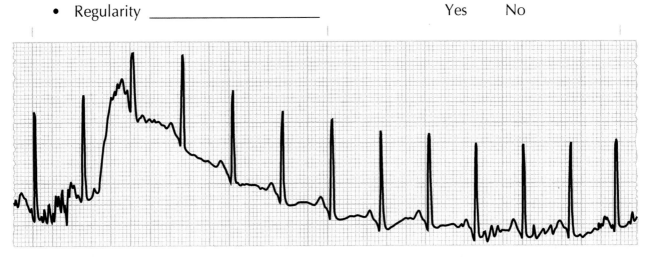

**40.** • Rate _____        Acceptable Quality Recording?

 • Regularity _____            Yes        No

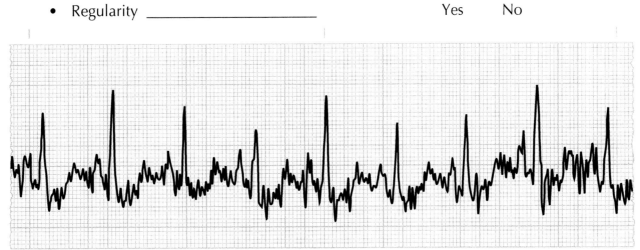

**Label the following diagram with the important anatomical landmarks.**

41.

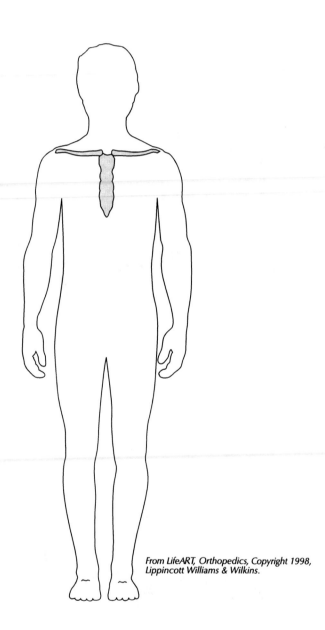

*From LifeART, Orthopedics, Copyright 1998, Lippincott Williams & Wilkins.*

Name_____

Date_____

**Draw in the positions of the chest leads.**

42.

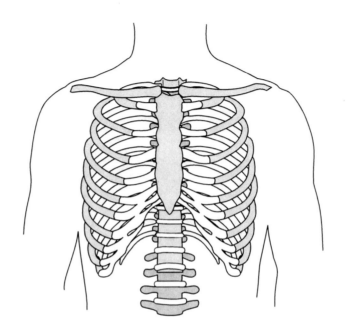

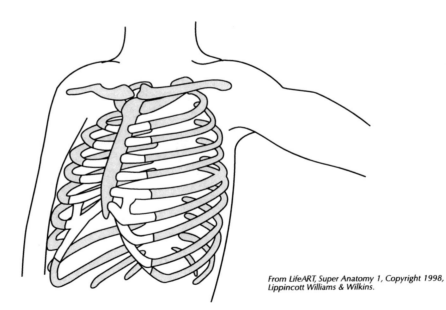

*From LifeART, Super Anatomy 1, Copyright 1998,
Lippincott Williams & Wilkins.*

# Chapter Six
# The Holter Monitor

## *Objectives*

After completing this chapter, you should be able to
do the following:

1. Define and correctly spell each of the key terms.

2. Describe the Holter monitor and discuss how it is similar
   and different from a 12-Lead ECG.

3. List three symptoms that may require testing with a
   Holter monitor.

4. List three conditions in which the use of a Holter monitor
   can be instrumental in determining a final diagnosis.

5. Describe the procedure for applying a Holter monitor
   to a patient.

6. Discuss how long the Holter is left on and why a diary
   is necessary.

7. Apply a Holter monitor to a fellow student.

## Key Terms

- bradycardia
- Holter monitor
- syncopal episode
- tachycardia

## Introduction

**Holter monitor:** a portable ECG recording machine that a patient wears which records the electrical activity of the heart continuously for 24 to 48 hours.

The **Holter monitor** is a portable monitoring device that provides a continuous ECG recording for a 24 to 48 hour period. It operates on the same principles as an ECG machine in that it records the electrical impulses of the heart muscle. It is different from an electrocardiograph in that the standard 12-Lead ECG records the heart's electrical activity for 12 views of the heart for a few seconds, whereas the Holter monitor records the heart's electrical activity for two to four views of the heart continuously over 24 to 48 hours.

## Indications for the Holter Monitor

The 12-Lead ECG provides vital information about the heart, but it displays only a few minutes worth of the heart's electrical activity. Frequently, the 12-Lead ECG is not able to capture abnormalities during the short period of time in which the test is taken. During a 12-Lead ECG the patient is lying quietly. Some heart abnormalities do not show up on an ECG unless the patient's activity places more demands on the heart. Because the Holter monitor records the heart rhythm over a longer period of time and under a variety of conditions, including activities of daily living, it is more likely to capture certain abnormalities than the standard 12-Lead ECG.

Usually the patient will undergo Holter monitoring as an outpatient, meaning that the monitor will be placed on the patient by a technician in a physician's (often a cardiologist's) office or clinic. The patient will then go home and resume normal activities. The idea is for the patient to participate in as many of his or her usual daily activities as possible in order to see which kinds of activities trigger heart abnormalities. The Holter monitor is very compact, about the size of a walkman or small radio. It is carried in a small case that has a shoulder strap or belt so that the monitor can be easily carried without interfering with the patient's activities.

The Holter monitor continuously records the heart rhythm and rate over a specified period of time, normally 24 to 48 hours. The patient's cooperation is essential because he or she has to keep a diary of all his or her activities and any related symptoms. This diary is then correlated to the ECG recording to see if there is any relationship between the heart rhythm and any activities or reported symptoms. This can be an effective and powerful diagnostic tool that can directly determine how the physician treats the patient's condition.

The patient should be instructed to write everything in the diary, including physical activities such as walking, eating, and driving, as well as emotional conditions such as being angry or anxious. The time of the activities should also be recorded. Any associated symptoms such as shortness of breath, chest pains, palpitations, light-headedness, dizziness, or faintness should also be recorded by the patient. Even the absence of symptoms should be noted. Sometimes symptoms may occur spontaneously, meaning that the symptoms may not be related to an activity, but occur while the patient is sitting quietly. All of this information should be noted in the diary. It is the technician's job to carefully explain this to the patient.

Continuous monitoring is useful in discovering ischemic changes and arrhythmias. Ischemic changes (poor blood flow to the heart) can cause symptoms of chest pain, shortness of breath, weakness, or arm pain.

Arrhythmias can be of several varieties. Arrhythmias are caused by two types of heartbeats. An unusually rapid heartbeat is called **tachycardia**, and an unusually slow heartbeat is called **bradycardia**. A discussion of the classifications and descriptions of arrhythmias can be found in Chapters Eight and Nine. For now, it is important to understand that in some situations tachycardias and bradycardias are dangerous, and in others they are not. For example, the heart beats fast during exercise. Tachycardia resulting from exercise is normal and healthy. Abnormal tachycardias occur because of a defect in the heart. They can occur at any time and can be life-threatening. Tachycardias can cause weakness, light-headedness, chest pain, heart pounding, and palpitations. While we are asleep, our heart beats slowly; this bradycardia is normal. But, if the heart beats slowly during exercise or if it beats too slowly during rest, then this is not normal. This type of bradycardia can cause weakness, shortness of breath, or light-headedness. Tachycardias and bradycardias can be regular or irregular, depending on the type. Sometimes irregular heartbeats are experienced as an unusual pounding sensation in the chest. Sometimes tachycardias and rhythm irregularities are experienced as an unusual sensation in the throat, like a tremor or fluttering.

**tachycardia:** a pulse rate above 100 beats per minute.

**bradycardia:** a pulse rate below 60 beats per minute.

**syncopal episode:** a fainting spell.

If a patient experiences a **syncopal episode**, then a Holter monitor can be useful in determining whether or not the cause lies within the heart. Very slow heart rates or very fast heart rates can cause syncopal episodes. Examining the Holter recording, the recorded activities, and related symptoms can provide useful information in determining if the primary cause of the syncopal episode was the heart.

The Holter recording is made on a magnetic tape, not on to paper. The record is initially read by a computer program, then it is reviewed by a technician, and then it is examined by the cardiologist. The heart rate and rhythm are determined, and abnormalities in the heart rate and rhythm are recorded. ECG changes that indicate ischemia are recorded. Tachycardias, bradycardias, and irregular heart rhythms are examined and classified. Abnormalities of the recording are correlated with activities and symptoms noted in the diary. All of this information is vital in assisting the physician with the formulation of an accurate diagnosis and determination of the best treatment.

After a patient receives surgical and/or medicinal treatment for the condition, then a Holter monitor might be used again to determine the effectiveness of the treatment.

## The Holter Monitor

The Holter monitor measures about four inches by six inches and weighs about two pounds. It has cables and lead wires similar to those on the electrocardiograph. The ends of the cables have attachments, either snaps or clips, that attach firmly to sensors on the patient's chest. The machine is carried in a small case for protection and convenience. It can be attached to a strap that can be worn over the shoulder, or it can be held in place by a belt secured around the patient's waist. It is designed to accompany the patient throughout his or her usual activities throughout the 24 to 48 hour period. The patient should be cautioned not to get the machine or cables wet; therefore, the patient should not take a bath or shower while wearing the Holter monitor.

Batteries power the Holter monitor. They are contained in a special battery compartment within the Holter monitor. The patient should be given backup batteries and instructed in how to change the batteries if they fail during the monitoring period. The monitor may beep or an indicator light may turn on to signal that the batteries need to be changed. New batteries should always be placed in the machine before each new recording session.

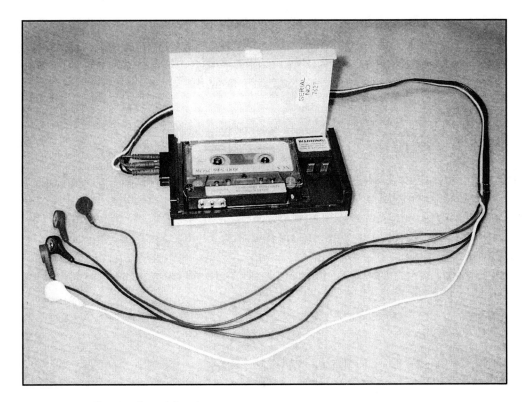

*Figure 6-1: The Holter Monitor*

Patients are not allowed to activate or deactivate the Holter monitor. A nurse or technician turns on the monitor using a switch that is located inside the box. The box is closed and put in a carrying case before the patient is allowed to take the monitor home.

When the machine is turned on, the electrical signals from the heart are transferred from the sensors on the surface of the skin to the machine. Instead of being printed onto ECG paper, the electrical signals are recorded onto a cassette tape inside the monitor. It would physically be impossible to record up to 48 hours worth of the heart rhythm directly onto ECG paper, but the tape is able to record continuously for 24 to 48 hours and save all of the ECG waveforms for that period. When the test is completed, the tape is processed by a computer, which reads and tallies the heart rate, rhythm, and all abnormal beats. A technician reviews the computer interpretation, and then the cardiologist makes the final interpretation and diagnosis. The heart's electrical information also can be printed out onto ECG paper, but usually only significant parts, such as runs of tachycardia or unusual heartbeats will be printed.

The Holter monitor is not able to record all 12 leads of the standard ECG. Usually, only two or three different leads are recorded. Typically a limb lead and a V lead are used, such as Leads II and $V_1$. If a third lead is used it may be another V lead, such as $V_6$, or a limb lead, such as Lead III.

## Lead Positions

The cables and lead wires are attached to one end of the Holter monitor case by plugging the metal prongs into the appropriate receptor site. The wires and receptors are usually color-coded in order to aid in the correct placement. There are three to six lead wires, depending on the type and age of the recorder used. Because the purpose of the Holter is to capture the heart rhythm during the daily living, the patient must have enough freedom of movement to maintain his or

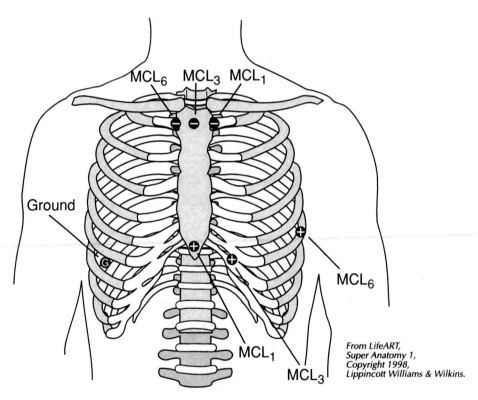

From LifeART,
*Super Anatomy 1,*
*Copyright 1998,*
*Lippincott Williams & Wilkins.*

For $MCL_1$, the negative sensor is placed below the clavicle just to the left of the manubrium, the positive sensor is placed below the sternum, at the xyphoid process. For $MCL_3$, the negative sensor is placed just over the manubrium, the positive sensor is placed approximately two inches away from the sternum at the border of the rib cage. For $MCL_6$, the negative sensor is placed below the clavicle just to the right of the manubrium, the positive sensor is at the level of the 6th rib in the midaxillary line. The ground sensor is placed on the right side of the chest.

*Figure 6-2: Example of Holter Monitor Chest Lead Placement*

her usual activities while being tested. To preserve this freedom of movement, the sensor positions for Holter monitoring are modified slightly from the standard 12-Lead ECG positions, these leads are referred to as *Modified Chest Leads*, or MCL$_x$. A ground sensor common to all leads is usually placed on the lower right portion of the torso.

For MCL$_1$, the positive sensor is placed at the V$_1$ position, 4th intercostal space at the right sternal border. In some monitoring systems, the positive electrode for a modified V$_1$ is placed at the bottom of the sternum, over the xyphoid process. The placement may vary depending on the equipment and manufacturer involved. Like V$_1$, MCL$_1$ is looking at the anterior, or front, portion of the heart.

Similarly, V$_3$ and V$_6$ can be modified. For a modified V$_3$, the negative electrode is placed directly over the manubrium. The positive electrode is placed on the left side of the chest approximately two inches from the left sternal border at the level of the 5th rib, or slightly lower at the edge of the rib cage.

With a modified V$_6$, the negative sensor is placed below the clavicle and to the right of the manubrium. The positive sensor is placed at the level of the 5th intercostal space at the midaxillary line. The positive sensor may also be placed slightly lower, at the 6th rib. Again, exact placement and modification may vary between institutions and manufacturers used.

Leads II and III may also be used in Holter monitoring; they are modified only slightly from the 12-Lead ECG position. Remember, during a 12-Lead ECG, the position of the sensors for Lead II is right arm negative and left leg positive, and Lead III is left arm negative and left leg positive. The patient's activities would be hampered to have sensors and wires attached directly to the limbs during the time that the monitor is worn. Also, the frequent motion of the limbs might cause interference (**artifacts**) in the electronic recording. Remember, artifacts are extra waves in the ECG tracing that hide the underlying electrical activity of the heart and make it difficult to read the final recording. To minimize the interference of the limb motion and to allow for free movement during activities, the sensors are placed on the torso near the joints. For Lead II the positive sensor is placed on the left lower part of the torso and the negative sensor is placed on the right upper arm at the shoulder joint. In Lead III the positive sensor is placed on the left lower part of the torso and the negative sensor is placed on the left upper arm at the shoulder joint.

The combination of leads used will vary by institution and manufacturer. Be sure that you have clear instructions from the institution for which you work as to which leads are commonly used and how they are to be modified for the Holter monitor. Frequent combinations are: Leads II, III, and $V_1$ ($MCL_1$); Leads II, $V_1$ ($MCL_1$), and $V_6$ ($MCL_6$); or Leads $V_1$ ($MCL_1$), $V_3$ ($MCL_3$), and $V_6$ ($MCL_6$). In the unit or clinic where you are working there should be a standardized procedure, a diagram, and instructions readily available.

# Holter Monitor Testing

**Materials needed:**
- ✓ A Holter monitor
- ✓ A magnetic tape (reel-to-reel or cassette, depending on type of monitor)
- ✓ Batteries - size of battery will vary with models used
- ✓ Lead wires - 5 to 7 required depending on model
- ✓ Sensors - self-adhesive, with gel in center
- ✓ Alcohol swabs and gauze pads
- ✓ A carrying case with shoulder strap or belt
- ✓ Hypoallergenic tape
- ✓ A disposable razor (if needed)
- ✓ A patient diary

1. Procedural Step: Wash your hands.
   Reason: Standard Precaution.

2. Procedural Step: Explain the procedure and the equipment to the patient.
   Reason: If the patient understands the procedure as well as its purpose and usefulness, then the patient will be more cooperative and less frightened.

3. Procedural Step: Insert the batteries and the magnetic tape into the Holter monitor.
   Reason: Batteries power the monitor.

4. Procedural Step: Cleanse the patient's skin.
   Reason: Cleansing the skin promotes optimal conduction of the electrical current.

5. Procedural Step: Place the sensors on the chest: right shoulder (for right arm); left shoulder (for left arm); right lower torso (for right leg); left lower torso (for left leg); fourth intercostal space at the right sternal border; level of fifth intercostal space at the anterior axillary line; and/or fourth intercostal space at the left sternal border.
   Reason: Correct sensor placement is essential for accurate recording of the heart rhythm.

## Holter Monitor Testing (Cont.)

6. Procedural Step: Attach the lead wires to the sensor pads. They usually snap on. Make sure to attach the correct wire to the appropriate location. The lead wires will probably be labeled with RA (right arm), LA (left arm), RL (right leg), LL (left leg), $V_1$, $V_6$, G (ground), and they may be color coded. The labeling and color coding will vary with different models.
Reason: Correct lead placement is essential for accurate recording of the heart rhythm.

7. Procedural Step: Reinforce the sensors with hypoallergenic tape. Tape over the sensor and the lead connection to secure it. Sometimes it is helpful to loop the wire in order to further secure it.

Reason: If the leads fall off, then information will be not be recorded and the test may have to be repeated.

8. Procedural Step: Turn on the Holter monitor. The switch is usually inside the Holter box. Make sure that it is running and that the indicator light is on.
Reason: If the machine is not turned on, it will not record.

9. Procedural Step: Place the Holter monitor in the carrying case and attach it to the shoulder strap or belt for easy carrying. Show the patient how to adjust the belt or strap for comfort. Assist the patient in putting on his or her clothes.
Reason: To make it easy for the patient to carry the device around.

# Holter Monitor Placement

## Patient Preparation

As with all procedures, the patient needs to be informed of the intent and purpose of the Holter monitor test. Inform the patient about the duration of the test, the application of the monitor, and the importance of patient cooperation during the test.

The nurse or doctor may have already explained the purpose of the test to the patient, but the technician should reinforce the information and should be ready to answer any questions. Explain that a Holter monitor is a 24 to 48 hour monitoring system and that it is designed to detect abnormalities that do not show up on the standard ECG. Make it clear that the patient is to resume his or her usual lifestyle and is to be as active as possible. Stress the importance of resuming normal physical activity during the testing procedure. When increased demands are placed on the heart, such as during physical or mental stress, abnormalities may occur in the ECG waveform or rhythm. These abnormalities will then be recorded by the Holter monitor. The patient may walk, perform normal tasks (such as light housework or job duties), and participate in all other activities of daily living. Vigorous exercise, however, should be avoided by patients undergoing a Holter monitor procedure. Tell the patient to avoid activities that might disrupt the lead connections. The patient also may not shower, take a bath, or swim because the Holter equipment and leads should not become wet.

Give the patient a blank booklet for use as a diary, and explain the purpose of keeping a detailed account of all activities and any symptoms that may occur. All aspects of the patient's daily routine should be entered in the diary: meals, exercise, sexual activity, bowel movements, chores, time medications are taken, etc. It is equally important to record symptoms such as fatigue, chest pain, light-headedness, and palpitations when they occur.

Instruct the patient to protect the leads and sensors to prevent them from being disconnected. When sleeping, he or she should wear a loose-fitting shirt so that the leads are protected and will not inadvertently be pulled off during sleep. While awake, it will be necessary to wear loose-fitting, comfortable clothing so that the monitor and leads will not be disrupted. The monitor should be worn outside of the clothing on the belt or shoulder strap provided.

Show the patient the features of the Holter monitor and familiarize him or her with the belt or strap. Tell the patient that he or she should not open the monitor case, but that he or she should examine the monitor periodically to make

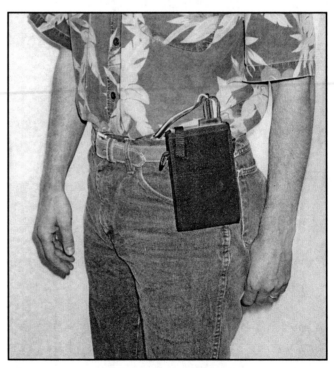

*Figure 6-3: Patient Wearing a Holter Monitor*

sure that it is running, the indicator light is on, and that all the cables and wires remain attached. It may also be necessary to show the patient how to change the batteries. Make sure the patient is provided with extra batteries before he or she leaves the premises.

| Time | Activity | Symptoms |
|------|----------|----------|
| 6 a.m. | Shower | None |
| 7 a.m. | Breakfast & medication | None |
| 8:15 a.m. | Walk to car | Chest pain |
| 11 a.m. | Walk up stairs | Short of breath |

Figure 6-4: A Holter Monitor Diary

## Skin Preparation

Skin preparation is the same as for the 12-Lead ECG. The areas on the chest that are designated for sensor placement should be cleansed with soap and water or an alcohol swab. The skin should then be dried by briskly rubbing the area with a gauze pad. The purpose is to remove dirt, sweat, and dead tissue. This cleansing provides a smooth surface that will enhance electrical conduction from the skin surface to the sensor. If the patient's chest is hairy, you may need to shave the area where the sensors will be placed. Ask the patient for permission to shave the chest.

# Chapter Summary

The Holter monitor is a portable device that provides a continuous record of the heart's activity over a 24 to 48 hour period. It is usually prescribed when a patient has experienced symptoms that the physician feels may be caused by a problem with the heart.

Patient preparation is very important to the success of this diagnostic procedure. The patient must thoroughly understand the necessity of recording, in a diary or log, certain activities of daily living and symptoms he or she may experience. The patient must also understand how to protect and maintain the Holter monitor during use and what activities should be avoided.

Proper application of the Holter monitor involves careful skin preparation and placement of the sensors as well as being sure it is working properly before the patient leaves the facility.

Name_____

Date_____

# Student Enrichment Activities

**Complete the following statements.**

1. The Holter monitor records the patient's heart rhythm for _____ to _____ hours onto a _____ _____.

2. The Holter monitor is used to diagnose _____ _____ and _____.

3. _____, _____, and _____ are symptoms that a patient may experience which require further testing with a Holter monitor.

4. The Holter is better able to catch abnormalities that the standard 12-Lead ECG may miss because it records the heart rhythm for a _____ period of time and it can record the heart rhythm when the patient is _____.

5. $MCL_1$ stands for _____ _____ _____ _____ and is a modification of _____ of the standard 12-Lead ECG.

6. Four leads that may be used with a Holter monitor are _____, _____, _____, and _____.

7. Limb leads are modified by placing the leads on the _____, near the _____.

8. The $V_3$ lead is modified by placing the negative sensor over the _____ and the positive sensor on the left side of the chest approximately two inches from the left _____ _____ at the level of the _____ rib.

9. The Holter tape is read by a computer, reviewed by a _____, and examined by a _____. The heart _____ and _____ are determined and abnormalities are recorded.

10. The _____ _____ _____is used to document patient activities and symptoms.

11. The skin is prepared by _____, _____, and, if required, _____.

12. Skin preparation enhances _____ _____.

**Complete the following exercises.**

13. Place a Holter monitor on a fellow student.

14. Explain the purpose of a Holter monitor and describe the procedure to a friend as if he or she was a patient and you were preparing to hook him or her up to a Holter monitor.

# Chapter Seven
# The Treadmill Stress Test

## *Objectives*

After completing this chapter, you should be able to
do the following:

1. Define and correctly spell each of the key terms.

2. Describe the information that can be obtained from a
   Treadmill Stress Test, or exercise ECG.

3. List three symptoms and conditions that may require further
   testing by a Treadmill Stress Test.

4. Discuss which conditions might make it unsafe to proceed
   with an exercise ECG.

5. Discuss symptoms that a patient may develop during a
   Treadmill Stress Test and the indications for prematurely
   stopping the testing.

6. Demonstrate how to take an accurate blood pressure
   reading.

7. Describe the role of the physician and/or nurse and the role
   of the technician during the Treadmill Stress Test.

8. Prepare and place electrodes on the patient in preparation
   for the exercise test.

## Key Terms

- blood pressure
- Persantine or dobutamine stress test
- target heart rate
- treadmill stress test (TMST)

# Introduction

**treadmill stress test (TMST):** a test in which a continuous 12-Lead ECG is recorded during a 15 to 20 minute exercise protocol on a treadmill to determine if heart disease is present; also called stress test, exercise ECG, or, simply, treadmill.

"Exercise ECG," "stress test," and **"treadmill stress test" (TMST)** are interchangeable terms. They all refer to exercising a patient to a specified target heart rate and monitoring the physiologic response throughout the test by running a continuous 12-Lead ECG. Increased demands are placed on the heart during exercise. So, the way in which the heart reacts to the stress of the exercise test can provide valuable information about the heart's health. It can be used as a screening tool for patients who have high risk factors for heart disease. It also can be used for patients with known heart disease to assess the severity of the disease and determine future treatment.

The exercise ECG can be used to determine the exercise tolerance of individuals with known heart disease, and can be used as a guide in formulating an exercise plan for that patient. Whereas the Holter monitor is used to determine the heart's response to routine activities, the TMST is used to determine the heart's response to maximum or near maximum exercise.

# Indications for a TMST

The TMST, or exercise ECG, is used as a screening test and as an evaluation tool. Many physicians recommend a TMST to assess the cardiovascular health of patients with known heart disease and those who are at high risk for heart disease. Some patients do not have any symptoms of heart disease until a heart attack threatens their life. Screening with a TMST may provide an indication of heart disease before a life-threatening event occurs. For a patient with known heart disease, the TMST can assess the severity of the heart disease and assist the medical team in determining if further testing is required.

When abnormalities show up on the TMST, treatments can be planned. If the TMST indicates heart disease, then an angiogram may be ordered to further assess the extent and severity of disease. Medications may be ordered and the patient may be advised to change his or her diet, lose weight, stop smoking, and start a regular exercise program.

A TMST is used as a diagnostic tool in patients with chest pain or shortness of breath. When a patient goes to the doctor's office and complains of chest pain, usually a standard 12-Lead ECG is done first. The standard 12-Lead is useful in determining if a myocardial infarction (heart attack) has occurred or is occurring, or if heart disease is present. In some cases, however, the heart may appear normal even if heart disease is present. A myocardial infarction (MI) is caused by complete blockages in the coronary arteries (blood vessels in the heart). These blockages prevent blood from getting to certain parts of the heart. The lack of blood causes some of the heart tissue to die and to release chemicals that interfere with the electrical pattern represented by the ECG, leading to ST segment elevation on the ECG. This is called an acute infarction pattern. Partial blockage of the coronary arteries will cause decreased blood flow to the heart muscle which results in ischemia. Ischemia occurs when the tissue is deprived of adequate supplies of oxygen and nutrients; however, since the tissue isn't completely shut off from the blood supply, tissue death does not occur. Ischemia is indicated on the ECG by ST segment depression. It is important to remember that ischemia is reversible, but infarction is not reversible.

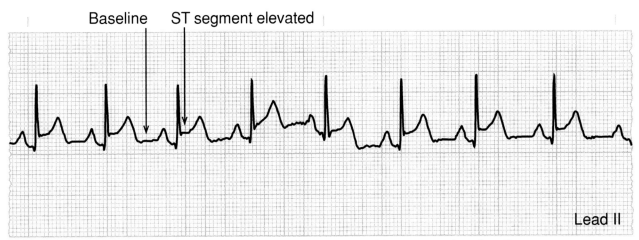

When the ST segment is higher than the baseline, this is called ST segment elevation. To be clinically significant, the elevation must be greater than one small box. The ST elevation in this example is about 2 1/2 small boxes.

*Figure 7-1: ST Segment Elevation*

During a resting ECG the ST segment may be normal, indicating that the blood supply to the heart is adequate for the resting state. The exercise treadmill test places increased demands on the heart. When the body is exercising, the heart has to work harder and more efficiently in order to pump enough blood to the exercising muscles. If partial blockages are present, then the heart will not get enough blood to the exercising muscles to meet the increased demands during the exercise state. An ST depression will occur if this is the case. This depression explains the premise of the TMST and how it can provide valuable information about the heart even when the resting ECG indicates everything is normal. The heart, under the stress of exercise, will show electrical abnormalities in the ECG that indicate decreased blood flow. Thus, the exercise ECG helps to diagnose coronary artery disease — a disease that causes blockages in the arteries supplying the heart muscle with blood.

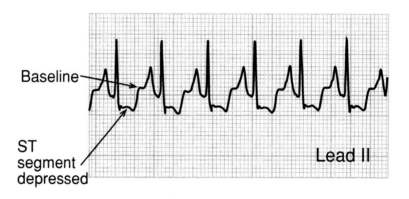

*Figure 7-2: ST Segment Depression*

The twelve leads of the standard ECG show different views of the heart and different areas of the heart muscle. Different leads represent the areas of heart muscle that are fed by specific coronary arteries. Therefore, abnormalities in a particular lead indicate the coronary arteries that may have disease and blockage. For example, Leads II and III are referred to as inferior leads, meaning that they view the inferior wall of the heart. Generally, these leads represent heart muscle fed by the right coronary artery. There are exceptions to this, but abnormalities in these leads give the physicians and nurses an indication of which blood vessels may be involved. An angiogram would have to be done in order to show exactly were the blockages exist.

An exercise ECG will show abnormalities in the heart rhythm. Sometimes, when the heart is stressed by exercise and ischemia occurs, the increased demands will cause irregularities in the heart rhythm. These abnormalities may be occasional irregularities or sustained tachycardias. The heart's normal response to exercise is to increase the heart rate, which increases the amount of blood pumped out to the rest of the body in response to the increased demand. But if severe ischemia is present, the decreased blood flow may cause abnormal tachycardias that can be life-threatening. A patient prone to have cardiac arrhythmias may require a TMST to determine if the arrhythmias are triggered or aggravated by exercise.

It is important to realize that abnormal tachycardia, persistent chest pain, and/ or ST elevation are serious occurrences. These occurrences can be life-threatening and require that the TMST be stopped immediately. This is why it is important to have emergency equipment nearby while a TMST is being performed. A nurse or physician will be monitoring the ECG recording and the patient during the test for this reason. A patient with severe heart disease is at risk for serious complications, so it is imperative that the patient's response to the test be monitored closely throughout the test.

The TMST may clearly show the presence of heart disease, or it can be inconclusive. If the test is inconclusive, this means that the results are difficult to read and the patient may require further testing to determine the presence or severity of heart disease. An inconclusive TMST usually means that an angiogram is required in order to see if blockages are present and to determine the degree of their severity.

The TMST cannot predict whether a patient will have a heart attack, but it can identify patients who have an increased risk of having a heart attack. The TMST is better at identifying male patients with an increased risk than it is at identifying female patients with an increased risk. Female patients have an increased number of "false positive" TMSTs. Women are more likely than men to have a TMST that indicates coronary artery disease when, in fact, they do not. The reason for this is unclear, but research is being done to attempt to explain it. The only way to definitively diagnose coronary artery disease is to perform an angiogram and directly look at the coronary arteries in order to determine if blockages are present.

TMSTs are frequently performed in physician's offices and hospitals as an important initial step in diagnosing coronary disease. The TMST is only part of the complete evaluation of a patient with suspected or known heart disease. The patient's medical history, physical exam, blood tests, and other tests give the physician the information necessary to effectively evaluate, diagnose, and treat the patient.

The treadmill stress test is an important tool in evaluating a patient's progress after a myocardial infarction (MI) or after cardiac surgery. Performance on the TMST can help the physician evaluate recovery and formulate a plan of care. After an MI or heart surgery most patients participate in a cardiac rehabilitation program to optimize their recovery. A patient's performance on the TMST serves as a guide to his or her exercise prescription and rehabilitation process. If a patient's initial performance on the treadmill demonstrates poor exercise tolerance, then he or she will need more time to reach the desired level of conditioning and complete the rehabilitation process.

During the TMST, the heart is pushed beyond the demands of routine activities. The "stress" part of the test refers to the demands placed on the heart during the course of exercise. During exercise the skeletal muscles demand more oxygen and nutrients, increasing the demands on the heart. The heart muscle also requires more oxygen and nutrients so it can beat harder and faster to deliver more blood to the rest of the body. The blood, carrying oxygen and nutrients, is delivered to the heart through the coronary arteries. If coronary artery disease is present, the delivery system is hampered by blockages in the blood vessels; the heart is not able to receive the increased flow of blood required to meet the increased needs of exertion. When the heart does not receive the required blood flow, symptoms such as chest pain, shortness of breath, or fatigue may occur. The TMST is useful in documenting how much exercise the patient can tolerate before experiencing symptoms of cardiac insufficiency. The TMST is a useful tool in determining future treatment.

## Contraindications for a TMST

There are conditions a patient may have which would make having a TMST dangerous. If a patient has a dissecting aortic aneurysm (a weakness in the wall of the aorta), a stress test should not be attempted. A patient with such a condition would be at a high risk to bleed or tear the aneurysm. Similarly, patients with irritation in or around the heart (myocarditis or pericarditis), uncontrolled hypertension, or untreated **congestive heart failure**, would not be candidates for a TMST because the demands placed on the heart may create severe respiratory distress. When these conditions are resolved or controlled a TMST may be performed. The presence of uncontrolled arrhythmias or unstable angina are also reasons a patient should not undergo this test. Heart attack patients should not undergo a TMST for 10 days to two weeks following the MI.

Having occasional bouts of arrhythmia or chest pain is different from experiencing continuous or uncontrolled symptoms. A patient should never be put on a treadmill if his or her baseline condition demonstrates arrhythmias or chest pain. Before having a TMST, the patient must have a baseline ECG, a thorough history, and physical exam by a cardiologist. These items are necessary to ensure that the patient's condition indicates the need for a TMST and that the patient will not be subjected to undue risk during the exercise test.

If proper precautions are not taken and the patient is exercised beyond the heart's capability to compensate for the increased demands placed on the heart, then the patient may develop severe chest pain, uncontrolled tachycardia, or even irreparable damage to the heart. Obviously, these situations are to be avoided as they may result in life-threatening conditions. However, the TMST, when properly performed, involves little risk to the patient.

## Patient Instruction

Prior to scheduling the test, a complete physical exam should be performed by a physician or nurse practitioner. This, along with a complete history of the patient, should reveal any contraindications to the test such as those already described.

Usually, the TMST is arranged days or weeks ahead of time. The test should be explained to the patient so that he or she understands the purpose and procedure of the test. The patient is instructed to prepare for the test by adjusting his or her routine activities for a few hours before the test in order to ensure optimum performance on the treadmill. Patient instructions include the following:

- Refrain from smoking for several hours before the test.
- Get a good night's sleep prior to the test and avoid strenuous physical activity for 8 to 12 hours before the test.
- Avoid alcohol and beverages containing caffeine. They can affect or alter the patient's performance.
- Avoid food for 3 to 4 hours before the test. Consume only light meals if you are hungry prior to this period on the day of the test. If a heavy meal is consumed just prior to the test, then the blood flow will be diverted to the stomach in order to digest the food and less blood will be available to the heart. Undigested food in the stomach may decrease exercise tolerance and increase the possibility of angina during the test.

The patient should be encouraged to wear clothing that does not restrict movement and is appropriate for exercise. Loose-fitting clothing, such as a jogging suit, and exercise shoes will make the patient comfortable and allow him or her to move freely.

## Exercise ECG Equipment

The exercise ECG is performed on a treadmill that is specially adapted for exercise stress testing. To make it possible for a technician to monitor the patient's progress during the test, the treadmill is connected to a computer and an ECG machine with a printer. A keyboard, which allows patient information to be entered into the database, and software, which contains the instructions for the computerized test (**protocols**) complete the treadmill apparatus. There are a variety of different models in use, but each model is different. The following is a general description of the way in which an exercise ECG treadmill works.

The treadmill apparatus is designed to gradually challenge the patient. The test starts out at a slow pace and low grade, or incline. The speed and incline are gradually increased, thereby increasing the patient's work load. There are different methods of progressing the speed and incline, called protocols. Experts have developed a variety of protocols and different cardiologists prefer different methods. Offices or institutions that perform TMSTs may use one or two different protocols and adapt them as necessary. The ECG technician will need to be familiar with all the different protocols used by his or her place of employment. Several protocols may be pre-programmed into the treadmill's computer. The computer will give the operator a choice of protocols. When a protocol is selected, the treadmill will increase the patient's work load automatically. Usually, the speed will increase from 1.5 to 6.0 miles per hour over an average 20 minute exercise period. The speed increases at a rate of about 0.9 miles per hour every 3 minutes. Similarly, the incline will increase progressively (from a 10% grade to a 22% grade) over the same 20 minute period.

The ECG machine that is connected to the treadmill has a viewing screen and a printer. The ECG machine will print the standard 12-Lead ECG continuously throughout the duration of the test.

## Additional ECG Equipment

Several other pieces of equipment are required for the TMST in addition to the treadmill apparatus. For example, a chart that displays the "Scale of Perceived Exertion" must be easily seen by the patient while on the treadmill. The nurse or doctor will refer to the chart during the exercise test, and periodically ask the patient to rate his or her exertion. The scale is numbered from 1 - 20. Next to each number is a statement describing a level of exertion. The statement next to number 1 refers to the exertion a person feels sitting in a chair, and the statement next to number 20 reflects maximal exertion. Numbers under 10 reflect light exertion, numbers 11 - 15 reflect moderate exertion, and numbers 16 - 20 reflect heavy exertion. Throughout the test, the nurse or doctor will ask the patient how he or she feels and request that the patient assign a number that accurately describes his or her feeling of exertion. It is important for those administering the test to have an accurate idea of how hard the patient is working and the patient's perception of that work. The patient may feel that he or she is working "hard" or "very hard," but should not feel like they are exercising to maximal capacity. Those monitoring the test should use subjective data (what the patient says) as well as objective data (how the patient looks, vital signs, etc.) when assessing how the patient is tolerating the testing procedure.

A blood pressure cuff and a stethoscope are essential pieces of equipment for an exercise ECG. The patient's blood pressure must be monitored frequently during the test. The blood pressure is an indicator of how hard the patient's heart is working in response to the activity.

An examination table or couch should also be nearby so that the patient may lie down during the recovery period, or if he or she has difficulties during the test, such as chest pain, they should also be allowed to lie down and rest.

## Emergency Equipment

Emergency equipment must be in the same room or close by while a TMST is being performed. Emergency equipment and medications are standardized and kept together on a cart, often called a crash cart. It is designed and organized for quick access and easy use.

On the top of the cart is a cardiac monitor and defibrillator pack. It is important to make sure that the monitor/defibrillator combination is plugged in, fully charged, and ready for use. If a life-threatening heart rhythm occurs during the TMST, then the defibrillator is used to shock the heart back into a normal rhythm. Lead cables and electrodes should also be attached to the monitor and ready for use. Gel pads or conductive gel should be on the top of the cart for use with the defibrillator. A suction machine and tubing should also be on top of the cart. In addition, an oxygen tank should be readily available as well as an oxygen mask, a bag valve and mask (used to force air into a patient that is not breathing), and oxygen tubing. The tank should be checked frequently to ensure that enough oxygen is available, if needed.

Medications that slow and regulate the heartbeat and intravenous (IV) fluids and tubing are stored in the drawers of the cart. When these medications are needed, the physician or nurse is responsible for starting the IV and giving the appropriate medications. An extra blood pressure cuff and stethoscope should also be on the cart. Other emergency equipment on the cart includes syringes, blood drawing equipment, and various tubes and catheters.

## Patient Preparation

When a patient first enters the testing room he or she may feel overwhelmed by the equipment and the testing process. Reassure the patient and make him or her feel as comfortable as possible. Explain that the patient needs to alert the nurse, physician, or technician immediately if he or she begins to experience chest pain or pressure, arm pain, or any other sensation that the patient may recognize as heart pain or angina. Orient the patient to the room. Explain the purpose of the equipment in order to relieve his or her fears. Point out the chart that describes perceived work effort. Explain the purpose of the chart, and that the chart will be referred to during the test to gauge the patient's response to the exercise test.

Outline the testing procedure so that the patient will know what to expect. Describe how the treadmill works, and instruct him or her in how to step onto the machine. Be sure the patient understands that the machine will gradually increase in speed and grade every few minutes. Inform the patient that this test is intended to make the heart work hard and that it will be a demanding workout. Make it clear to the patient that if at any time he or she develops chest pain, severe shortness of breath, light-headedness, or dizziness the physician, nurse, or technician should be informed immediately. If at any time during the test, the patient feels his or her limit has been reached, he or she should speak up and notify the nurse.

Lead placement is similar to that of a 12-Lead ECG. Limb leads, augmented limb leads, and chest leads are used during the TMST. The sensors for the limb leads will need to be placed on the torso instead of on the limbs, because the leads will inhibit free movement by the patient if they are placed on the arms and legs. Otherwise, the movement will create artifacts and make it difficult to read the ECG.

Place the right arm sensor at the right shoulder below the clavicle. Place the left arm sensor near the left shoulder below the clavicle. The right leg sensor is placed on the right side of the chest at the lowest palpable rib on the anterior axillary line. Similarly, the left leg sensor is placed on the left side of the chest at the lowest palpable rib on the anterior axillary line. These positions will accommodate the need for free movement and yet provide the proper views for the 12-Lead ECG. Place the V leads as for the standard 12-Lead ECG on the anterior chest. Check placement by using the landmarks of the ribs and sternal border as described previously. $V_1$ is at the 4th intercostal space at the right sternal border; $V_2$ is at the 4th intercostal at the left sternal border; $V_4$ is at the 5th intercostal at the midclavicular line; $V_3$ is between $V_2$ and $V_4$; $V_5$ is at the left anterior axillary line at the level of the 5th intercostal space; $V_6$ is also at the level of the 5th intercostal space, but at the left midaxillary line.

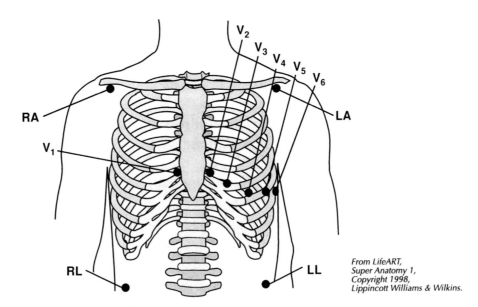

*From LifeART, Super Anatomy 1, Copyright 1998, Lippincott Williams & Wilkins.*

*Figure 7-3: TMST Lead Placement*

Skin preparation is similar to that previously described in earlier chapters. Cleanse the patient's skin where the sensors are to be placed. Use soap and water or alcohol swabs. Shave the patient's chest as necessary.

# Determining a Patient's Target Heart Rate

**target heart rate:**
the heart rate an
individual should
reach to achieve
optimal aerobic
exertion without
chest pain, SOB,
or ECG abnor-
malities.

The **target heart rate** is the heart rate the patient should achieve during the exercise test. It is important for the patient to exercise to near maximal capacity, because the stress placed on the heart during near maximal exertion is the condition that is being examined. The heart rate reflects the extent of the stress that is being placed on the heart, or the level of the heart's exertion. The physical stress, or demands, placed on the heart during the exercise test stimulates physiological changes in the healthy heart and its surrounding tissues. For instance, in response to increased demands placed on the heart, the blood vessels will dilate, increasing blood flow to and from the heart. In a heart with disease, blood vessels cannot dilate sufficiently and the increased demands for oxygen and nutrients in the heart are not met, creating symptoms of stress to the heart, such as chest pain, shortness of breath, or fatigue. The extent of exertion and increased demand on the heart is estimated by the heart rate. Preprinted reference charts may be used to determine the target heart rate, or a formula may be used.

A patient's target heart rate is based on his or her age. To determine the patient's target heart rate, subtract the patient's age from 220 to get the theoretical maximum heart rate for the patient. Then, calculate 90% of that number and round it off to get the target heart rate for that individual. For example, the target heart rate for a 37 year-old patient would be calculated in the following way:

1. Calculate the patient's maximum heart rate.
   220-(the patient's age) = patient's maximum heart rate
   220-37 = patient's maximum heart rate
   183 = patient's maximum heart rate

2. Then, multiply the maximum heart rate by 90%.
   patient's max. heart rate x 0.90 = patient's target heart rate
   183 x 0.90 = patient's target heart rate
   164.7 = patient's target heart rate

3. Round off the target heart rate to the nearest whole number.
   165 = patient's target heart rate (rounded off)

As you can see from the example, for a 37 year-old to achieve optimal aerobic exertion, he or she would have to attain a heart rate of 165 beats per minute. If the target heart rate is achieved without chest pain, severe shortness of breath, or ECG abnormalities, then the patient is probably free of heart disease or has minimal heart disease. If chest pain or ECG abnormalities occur, then heart disease is most likely present and further tests will be required.

If a patient is elderly, feeble, weak, or disabled from another disease process, then it may be unrealistic to expect the patient to reach the target heart rate. In this case, the doctor or nurse may use a lower target heart rate. A TMST that uses a lower target heart rate is called a sub-maximal treadmill stress test. Alternatively, a **Persantine** or **dobutamine stress test** may be ordered. In these two tests a drug (Persantine or dobutamine) is given to the patient to increase the heart rate artificially, without exercise. The increased heart rate will stress the heart in a similar way as the increased heart rate of exercise. As in the exercise test, chest pain, shortness of breath, and ECG abnormalities are the criteria for determining a positive test, or the presence of disease.

**Persantine (or dobutamine) stress test:** a procedure used when a patient is unable to physically perform the stress test and the medication, Persantine or dobutamine, is given to the patient in order to artificially raise the heart rate and see how the heart performs when stressed.

# Roles of Healthcare Professionals

The treadmill stress test is carried out by two healthcare professionals. The work is divided into two roles that must be fulfilled. One of the roles is carried out by a physician or nurse and the second is carried out by a technician. If a physician is not assisting with the test or is not in the room where the test is being performed, then a physician must be available in the office in case of an emergency.

The role of the technician and the role of the physician or nurse may vary and even overlap in different facilities. Usually, the role of the technician is to attach the patient to the monitoring equipment, enter patient information into the treadmill computer, assist in obtaining blood pressure readings at intervals during the test, and assess the patient's other vital signs, skin color, and level of exertion. (The procedure for obtaining a blood pressure reading follows the procedure for administering the treadmill stress test.) The technician also will be responsible for explaining the procedure and the "scale of perceived exertion" to the patient.

The role of the physician or the nurse is to monitor the continuous ECG recording, observe for ECG abnormalities, assess the patient's condition during the exercise and recovery period, and watch for signs that may indicate the patient is exceeding his or her exercise limitations. If the patient has severe ECG abnormalities, or if the patient experiences severe chest pain or shortness of breath, then the test may be stopped prematurely. The physician or nurse assesses the ECG and the patient's condition before each increase in speed and grade. He or she warns the patient that a change in speed will occur and assesses whether the patient is ready for that increase.

Prior to the increase in speed, the technician will check the blood pressure. The physician or nurse will enter the blood pressure, perceived exertion rating, and any symptoms the patient is experiencing into the treadmill computer. The chart of perceived exertion should be easily seen by the patient so he or she can refer to it throughout the exercise test.

The speed of the treadmill can be adjusted manually, or the timing may be preprogrammed. In either case, the patient should be assessed for his or her response to the exercise prior to the increase. The patient should also be warned about the increase.

# Treadmill Stress Test

**Materials needed:**

✔ sensors

✔ cables

✔ a treadmill

✔ emergency equipment

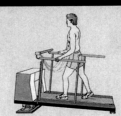

*From LifeART, Healthcare 1, Copyright 1998, Lippincott Williams & Wilkins.*

1. Procedural Step: Escort the patient into the treadmill stress test room and describe the purpose of the equipment and the procedure to the patient.
Reason: To relieve the patient's anxiety.

2. Procedural Step: Turn the computer on and use the keyboard to enter the patient's name, age, medical record number, and other information. Check to make sure that the electrocardiograph is loaded with adequate paper. Check the protocol programmed into the machine and make sure that the correct protocol is selected.
Reason: To ensure that the correct exercise protocol is used for the patient.

3. Procedural Step: Obtain a baseline (resting) blood pressure, heart rate, and respiratory rate.
Reason: A baseline is necessary to compare the testing and recovery vital signs to the resting vital signs.

4. Procedural Step: Have the patient lie down. Prepare the patient's skin for sensor placement. Cleanse and shave as required.
Reason: To ensure proper conduction of the electrical current.

5. Procedural Step: Place the sensors in the locations you would use to obtain a 12-Lead ECG, with the limb sensors appropriately modified on the torso for the exercise test.

Reason: A 12-Lead recording is required for complete evaluation of the heart.

6. Procedural Step: Attach the correct leads to the placed sensors.
Reason: To obtain an accurate reading.

7. Procedural Step: Run a baseline or resting ECG.
Reason: A baseline is necessary to compare with the testing ECG.

8. Procedural Step: The nurse or physician will examine the resting ECG. If there are no severe abnormalities and the patient is free of chest pain, the test will continue.
Reason: Severe abnormalities may indicate that it is not safe to proceed with the TMST.

9. Procedural Step: Have the patient stand. Make sure that the blood pressure cuff and sensors stay in place as the patient rises. You may have to tape the sensors in place. Put the cable over the patient's shoulder to prevent it from getting in the way as he or she exercises.
Reason: To ensure that contact with the leads is not lost during the test.

10. Procedural Step: Turn the treadmill on at the slowest speed. Describe how to step onto the treadmill. The patient should first straddle the treadmill, then quickly place one foot at a time onto the moving belt of the treadmill. You may

# Treadmill Stress Test (Cont.)

have to demonstrate this to the patient. Railings on either side of the treadmill assist the patient in getting on and maintaining balance. When the test is in progress the patient should be instructed to let go of the railings.
*Reason:* To maintain the patient's safety and to ensure the accuracy of the test.

11. Procedural Step: The nurse or physician will monitor the heart rhythm on the screen and on the printout as the patient exercises. The machine will increase in speed and grade every few minutes. The nurse or physician will inform the patient of the increases and ask the technician to retake the blood pressure just prior to the speed changes, every 3 to 5 minutes. The technician will observe the patient for fatigue or weakness, and watch for signs that the patient (especially an elderly patient) may stumble and fall. The technician should have the patient refer to the scale of perceived exertion and rate his or her exertion according to the ratings on the scale.
*Reason:* To ensure the safety of the patient and the accuracy of the procedure.

12. Procedural Step: The process continues until the treadmill has increased to the maximum speed and grade prescribed by the protocol. Completion of the protocol takes about 15 to 20 minutes. After the first 5 or 10 minutes the patient should have reached the target heart rate and be exercising aerobically. Continue to check the blood pressure every 3 to 5 minutes. The patient's blood pressure, symptoms, and perceived exertion are entered into the treadmill computer by a nurse or technician (assigned tasks vary by facility).

*Reason:* The blood pressure, symptoms, and perceived exertion are correlated with the ECG in final analysis.

13. Procedural Step: When the protocol is completed and the target heart rate has been achieved and maintained for 10 to 15 minutes, then the test is completed. The usual procedure is that the treadmill slows down and the patient continues to walk at a slow pace in order to cool down. Continue with blood pressure checks, assess how the patient feels, and obtain the patient's rating for the perceived exertion. If a patient experiences pain or is too weak to go on, the test will be stopped before the target heart rate is reached.
*Reason:* A cool-down period after exercise is always important in order to allow the body to adjust to a different level of activity.

14. Procedural Step: After a few minutes of cool down, have the patient step off the machine and step over to the table or couch. Instruct him or her to lie down. Continue with blood pressure checks and other patient assessments until the heart rate, blood pressure, and ECG return to baseline or resting state. The nurse or doctor will continue to monitor the ECG for abnormalities.
*Reason:* When the blood pressure, heart rate, and ECG return to baseline, the patient is considered to have recovered from the test.

# Blood Pressure

A patient's **blood pressure** is a source of important information for the primary healthcare provider and is an essential element of the treadmill test. A detailed description of the procedure for obtaining a blood pressure reading appears at the end of this chapter; however, an overview of the concept will assist in understanding the steps of the procedure.

**blood pressure:** the pressure of the blood exerted against the arteries.

A blood pressure reading is obtained by applying pressure to the brachial artery, which restricts the flow of blood through the artery. This restricted blood flow can be heard through a stethoscope as a light tapping sound. Using this tapping sound as a guide, the blood's pressure against the artery wall is measured at specific moments.

A stethoscope is a listening device that consists of a round diaphragm that transmits sounds through a tube to the earpieces. When obtaining a blood pressure reading, the diaphragm of the stethoscope is placed over the brachial artery, which is located on the inner aspect of the upper arm near the bend of the elbow joint. The stethoscope is used to listen for the flow of blood through the brachial artery.

The instrument used to create the pressure on the brachial artery and measure the pressure of the blood exerted against the artery is called a **sphygmomanometer**, or a blood pressure cuff. A sphygmomanometer consists of a cloth or nylon cuff that has an expandable rubber bladder inserted into a pocket in the fabric. The bladder is attached to a pressure gauge, a valve, and a hand pump or bulb. The cuff is wrapped around the patient's upper arm and fastened, usually with a velcro strip.

With the stethoscope in place, the cuff of the sphygmomanometer is pumped up until the tapping sound of blood flowing through the brachial artery cannot be heard through the stethoscope. When the tapping sound stops the brachial artery is fully occluded, meaning that blood is unable to flow through the artery. The valve is then slowly opened, decreasing the air pressure in the cuff to the point where blood is able to flow through the artery again. The technician listens for the return of the tapping sound in the artery and notes the number indicated on the gauge as soon as that sound is heard. The number that corresponds to this first tapping sound is the **systolic** blood pressure and represents arterial pressure during contraction of the heart. The technician continues to release pressure from the cuff in a slow and controlled manner until the tapping sound can no longer be heard, indicating that the artery is fully open. When the tapping stops, the number indicated on the gauge during the final tapping sound is noted. This number is the **diastolic** pressure and represents arterial pressure during relaxation of the heart.

The blood pressure is recorded as a fraction with the systolic number first, or on top, followed by the diastolic number on the bottom (eg, 120/80). The usual range of a resting blood pressure is 90-140 mm Hg for the systolic reading and 60-90 mm Hg for the diastolic reading.

During exercise the blood pressure will be elevated because the heart is working harder to get blood to the exercising muscles. After exercising, the blood pressure will gradually return to the normal range.

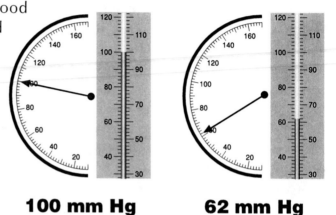

**100 mm Hg          62 mm Hg**

*Figure 7-4: Examples of Sphygmomanometer Readings*

The accuracy of the blood pressure reading is dependent on several factors: proper size of the sphygmomanometer; movement and cooperation of the patient; lack of excessive noise and distractions; the emotional state of the patient; disease processes; trauma; and a properly working sphygmomanometer and stethoscope. To get a proper reading, the width of the blood pressure cuff should cover approximately 3/4 the size of the patient's upper arm. A false high reading can be obtained if the cuff is too narrow, and a false low reading can be obtained if the cuff is too wide. Pediatric and infant cuffs are available for children and infants.

Accurate measurement of a blood pressure requires practice. The values are measured in millimeters of mercury, abbreviated as mm Hg. There are three main types of blood pressure sphygmomanometers. The mercury sphygmomanometer contains a large column of mercury (Hg). Each separate mark on the gauge, or manometer, represents 2 mm Hg. The aneroid sphygmomanometer does not contain a mercury column; it involves only a needle dial in which each line represents 2 mm Hg pressure. The third type is an electronic cuff. The cuff is placed on the patient's extremity; and an electronic machine will calculate the blood pressure. Make sure you are familiar with the proper operation of the machine before attempting to use it. Please note that blood pressure readings for newborns and infants require special instruction. Do not attempt to obtain a blood pressure on an infant without proper training.

There are many different factors that can affect blood pressure measurements:

- emotions (anger, fear)
- medications (prescribed or illegal)
- diet and weight
- stress (hospitalization, death, divorce, etc.)
- the patient's position

The position the patient is in during the blood pressure (BP) measurement may have a direct effect on the BP reading. Lying (supine), sitting, and standing blood pressure readings may vary slightly. If the variation is less than a 10 point change (10 mm Hg), then that is considered a normal variant. If the change in blood pressure is 10 points or more from one position to another, then this is considered an inappropriate BP response and must be investigated further. The term used for checking blood pressure in the lying, sitting, and standing position is called "orthostatic BP." Medications, hydration, and neurologic factors may contribute to an inappropriate blood pressure response to a position change.

Learning the normal limits of blood pressure will take time, but the ability to recognize changes in your patient's blood pressure values is an important part of your patient assessment skills.

# Auscultating a Blood Pressure

**Materials needed:**
- ✓ a stethoscope
- ✓ a sphygmomanometer (in the proper size for the patient)
- ✓ alcohol sponges
- ✓ gloves (if blood or other body fluids are present)

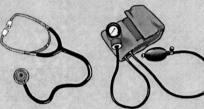

*From LifeART, Healthcare 1, Copyright 1998, Lippincott Williams & Wilkins.*

1. <u>Procedural Step:</u> Wash your hands and assemble the equipment.
   <u>Reason:</u> Standard Precaution.

2. <u>Procedural Step:</u> Clean the earpieces of the stethoscope with an alcohol sponge before using it.
   <u>Reason:</u> To protect against possible infection.

3. <u>Procedural Step:</u> Put on gloves if there is any blood or other body fluid present.
   <u>Reason:</u> Standard Precaution.

4. <u>Procedural Step:</u> Identify the patient.
   <u>Reason:</u> This confirms that you are assessing the correct patient.

5. <u>Procedural Step:</u> Explain the procedure to the patient using terms he or she will understand.
   <u>Reason:</u> This keeps the patient calm and provides the information necessary for the patient to give informed consent.

6. <u>Procedural Step:</u> Have the patient sit or lie down. Roll the patient's sleeve about 6 inches above the elbow. If the sleeve is too tight, remove the arm from the sleeve. Extend the arm, palm up, at heart level.

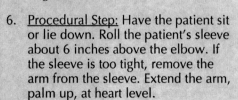

<u>Reason:</u> A sleeve that is too tight may compress the brachial artery and distort the results. If the arm is above heart level the reading may be incorrectly low.

7. <u>Procedural Step:</u> Palpate the brachial artery on the inner aspect of the elbow. Then place the blood pressure cuff smoothly and securely around the patient's arm about 2 inches above the bend in the elbow. Be sure the middle of the cloth-enclosed cuff is directly over the brachial artery on th inner aspect of the upper arm. If the cuff has an arrow to indicate right or left arm, the arrow should be placed over the brachial artery.
   <u>Reason:</u> The cuff should be tight enough to stay on, but not so tight as to be constricting. It should be high enough so that the stethoscope will not touch the cuff and cause extraneous sounds. By placing the center of the bladder of the cuff over the brachial artery you assure that the pressure is applied equally over the artery.

8. <u>Procedural Step:</u> Place the earpieces of the stethoscope in your ears with the tips pointing slightly forward. Avoid letting the tubes rub together.
   <u>Reason:</u> The forward position of the earpieces will make it easier to hear because they will be following the direction of the ear canal. The tubes should be hanging freely so extraneous sounds won't be heard.

# Auscultating a Blood Pressure (Cont.)

9. Procedural Step: Palpate the pulse at the brachial artery. Place the **diaphragm** of the stethoscope firmly over the point of maximal impulse (PMI).
Reason: Proper placement of the diaphragm will help you hear the sounds of the blood pressure.

10. Procedural Step: Hold the diaphragm in place with your nondominant hand, close the control valve and quickly squeeze the bulb with your dominant hand until you can no longer hear the pulse.
Reason: The range of 20 to 30 mm Hg is sufficient to be sure you have pumped the cuff high enough to accurately hear the systolic pressure. Inflating the rubber bladder in the cuff stops the flow of blood in the artery. The cuff is inflated quickly and smoothly to avoid congestion in the blood vessels.

11. Procedural Step: Slowly and steadily open the control valve at a rate of approximately 2 to 3 mm Hg per heartbeat. This will release the air in the cuff. Listen for the first clear, tapping sound. This is the systolic pressure. Notice the reading on the calibrated scale.
Reason: The systolic blood pressure represents the pressure against the walls of the arteries when the ventricles of the heart contract and blood surges through the aorta and pulmonary arteries.

12. Procedural Step: Continue to steadily deflate the cuff until the last sound is heard. This is the diastolic pressure.
Reason: The diastolic pressure refers to the point at which there is the least pressure in the arteries and occurs when the heart relaxes (diastole) before the next contraction (systole).

13. Procedural Step: Quickly release the rest of the air from the cuff and remove the cuff from the patient's arm. (Or leave the deflated cuff in place if frequent blood pressure readings are to be done.)
Reason: If left inflated, it will prevent circulation to the hand and arm.

14. Procedural Step: Immediately record the measurements obtained as a fraction, noting the time, arm used (right or left), and the patient's position (lying, sitting, or standing).
Reason: Charting immediately will ensure accuracy.

15. Procedural Step: Clean the earpieces and the diaphragm of the stethoscope with an alcohol sponge.
Reason: The equipment will be ready for use the next time.

16. Procedural Step: Remove your gloves if it was necessary to put them on.
Reason: Standard Precaution.

17. Procedural Step: Wash your hands before providing care to another patient.
Reason: Standard Precaution.

---

## Auscultating a Blood Pressure (Cont.)

Chart it like this, indicating which arm was used and whether the patient was sitting or lying down: BP=160/90 RA, sitting  meaning the blood pressure was 160 mm Hg systolic and 90 mm Hg diastolic, and the reading was taken on the right arm with the patient in a sitting position.

**Note:** When listening for the diastolic pressure, you will notice a change in the quality of the sounds before they completely disappear. Some physicians consider this change to be the first diastolic blood pressure. If you are asked to record this sound, chart it as follows: B/P 180/100/90. This would mean that the first sound you heard was 180 (systolic blood pressure), a change or muffled sound was noted at 100 (first diastolic sound), and the last sound you heard was at 90 (final diastolic pressure).

---

# Precautions

As stated earlier, there may be reasons to stop the test before the target heart rate is reached or before the preset increases of speed and incline are completed. If the patient develops chest pain that persists, severe shortness of breath, or if he or she requests to stop, then the test should be stopped. Severe elevation in blood pressure and certain ECG abnormalities also are signals to stop the test. In general, the nurse or physician will stop the test if the ECG shows signs of heart damage (ST elevation). The test will be continued if there are signs of ischemia, or decreased blood flow (ST depression), unless it is severe and/or the patient develops chest pain. If the patient complains of dizziness, then the test should be stopped. If the patient becomes pale, clammy, or **diaphoretic** (signs that the patient is in distress), then the test needs to be stopped. Another reason to discontinue the test is if the patient's heart rate becomes erratic or is much faster than his or her target heart rate.

# Chapter Summary

This chapter concludes the discussion about diagnostic tests covered in this book. The value of a TMST in diagnosing coronary heart disease is that it evaluates the ability of the heart to respond to the increased demands of exercise. If blockages in the coronary arteries are present, then the heart will not be able to get an appropriate level of blood flow during periods of increased demand such as exercise. Stress on the heart caused by exercise and increased demands will show up as ischemia, or decreased blood flow, on the ECG.

TMST involves the continuous 12-Lead ECG recording during the "stress" of exercise. Blood pressure and the patient's perceived exertion are monitored and recorded during and after exercise.

Explaining the procedure to the patient and preparing the patient for the test are important factors in obtaining accurate testing results. The sensors for the limb leads are placed on the torso (to avoid recording arm and leg movements) and the V leads are placed in the same location as a standard 12-Lead ECG. A cool-down period after the test is required for adequate patient recovery.

7-24

Name_____

Date_____

# Student Enrichment Activities

**Complete the following statements.**

1. The exercise ECG is also called the _____ _____
   _____ or _____ (initials).

2. One purpose of the exercise ECG is to diagnose and identify patients at risk for
   having _____ _____.

3. Another purpose of the TMST is to serve as a baseline test for patients recovering
   from a myocardial infarction or open heart surgery and who will participating in a
   _____ _____ program.

4. _____ _____ and _____ _____ _____
   are symptoms that may prompt a physician to order an exercise ECG.

5. The formula for determining target heart rate is _____ - _____ x
   _____.

6. The target heart rate is the heart rate an individual should reach to achieve
   _____ _____ _____ without chest pain, SOB,
   or ECG abnormalities.

7. If a patient is 70 his or her target heart rate will be _____.

8. The recovery, or cool down, period is the period of time it takes the _____
   _____, _____ _____, and _____ to return to
   _____, or resting state, after the exercise test.

9. The _____ of _____ _____ measures the patients' concept of how hard they feel that they are working when exercising on the treadmill.

10. The patient must have a baseline or resting _____ _____, _____ _____, and _____ _____ taken before performing the exercise test on the treadmill.

11. The role of the technician during the procedure includes (but is not limited to): taking the patient's _____ _____; entering _____ _____ into the treadmill computer; and assessing the patient's other vital signs, skin color, and _____ ____ _____.

12. The room in which the exercise ECG is done must have a _____ _____ in case complications occur.

13. Reasons to discontinue the exercise ECG include _____ _____, _____ _____ _____, and _____ _____.

14. A _____ is used in taking a blood pressure reading.

**Circle the correct answer.**

15. To prepare a patient for the exercise ECG he or she will be requested to refrain from:
    A. eating for 3 hours prior to the test.
    B. wearing comfortable loose fitting clothing.
    C. strenuous activity for 12 hours prior to the test.
    D. smoking for 2 hours prior to the test.
    E. A, C, and D.

Name_____

Date_____

16. An exercise ECG is contraindicated (not advised) for patients with:

    **A.** dissecting aortic aneurysm.

    **B.** heart failure or enlarged heart.

    **C.** uncontrolled hypertension.

    **D.** ulcers.

    **E.** A and C.

17. A doctor may decide to exercise a patient at a lower level if the patient:

    **A.** Is elderly.

    **B.** Has lung disease.

    **C.** Is too weak.

    **D.** Is an Olympic athlete.

    **E.** A, B, and C.

**Complete the following exercises.**

18. Calculate your own target heart rate.

    _____

    _____

    _____

19. On a separate sheet of paper, write the purpose and procedure of the exercise ECG in the same words you would use to explain the procedure to a patient if you were preparing him or her for the test.

**Write the sphygmomanometer readings in the spaces below.**

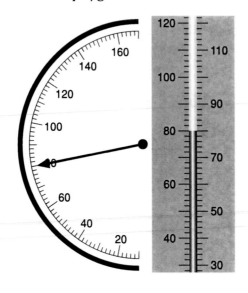

20. _____

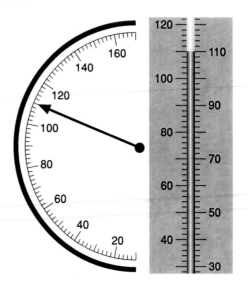

21. _____

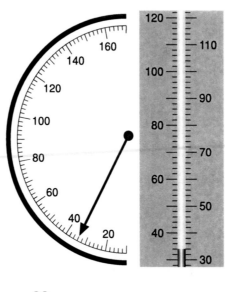

22. _____

# Chapter Eight
# Basics of Rhythm Interpretation

## *Objectives*

After completing this chapter, you should be able to
do the following:

1.  Define and correctly spell each of the key terms.

2.  Describe the requirements for normal sinus rhythm (NSR), including the rate and the rhythm, and the length of the waveforms.

3.  Describe how to examine the heart rhythm — including the analysis of the rate and the rhythm, and the measurement of the waveforms.

4.  Identify and properly measure components of the ECG waveform.

5.  State the normal duration for the PR interval and QRS complex.

6.  Describe two techniques for measuring waveforms.

7.  Identify normal sinus rhythm.

8.  Describe two variations of NSR.

# Key Terms

- calipers
- heart block
- normal sinus rhythm (NSR)

- sinus arrhythmia
- sinus bradycardia
- sinus tachycardia

# Introduction to Rhythm Analysis

Before beginning this chapter, it may be helpful to review the information in Chapter Four regarding the design and function of the ECG graph paper, characteristics of ECG waveforms, measurements of waveforms, and the components of a sinus rhythm. Although a brief review of these topics is included in this chapter, a thorough understanding of these concepts is vital to comprehension of the key elements of rhythm interpretation.

# ECG Graph Paper – A Review

It is important to remember the time intervals represented by the lines and squares on the graph paper. Time is represented along the horizontal lines of the paper. Remember that each small square represents 0.04 seconds and each large square represents 0.2 seconds. This information is essential in determining the length or duration of each waveform, as well as in calculating the heart rate.

Hash marks appear in a horizontal line along the top of the graph paper. The hash marks are set at intervals of three seconds. These marks are useful in estimating a patient's heart rate.

The vertical axis represents voltage. The taller the waveform, the more voltage it represents. Although voltage is important in the interpretation of a 12-Lead ECG, it is not a significant factor in rhythm analysis.

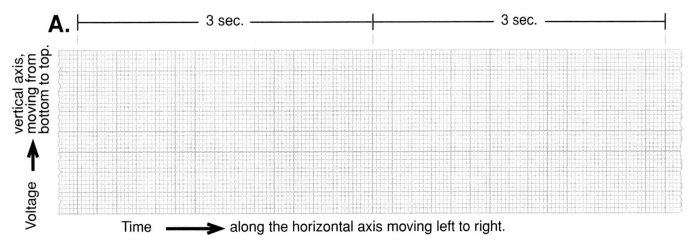

**A.** |——————— 3 sec. ———————|——————— 3 sec. ———————|

vertical axis, moving from bottom to top.

Voltage ↑

Time ——→ along the horizontal axis moving left to right.

Notice that the graph paper grid has heavy lines and lighter lines. The lighter lines create small boxes. The heavier lines create large boxes. Time is represented along the horizontal lines, moving from left to right. Moving from left to right from one light line to the next, equals 0.04 seconds. Moving from one heavy line to the next equals 0.20 seconds.

Hash marks on the top of the ECG paper help to mark time. The distance from one hash mark to the next represents 3 seconds; the distance from the first hash mark to a third hash mark represents 6 seconds, or $^1/_{10}$ of a minute. 15 large boxes take up the space between two hash marks (0.20 sec. X 15 = 3 sec.)

300 *large* boxes will span ONE MINUTE.

1500 *small* boxes will span ONE MINUTE.

Two large boxes, when traveling from bottom to top equals 1 mV (millivolt). While the measurement of time is essential to working with ECGs on an elementary level, measurement of voltage is more important on the advanced level.

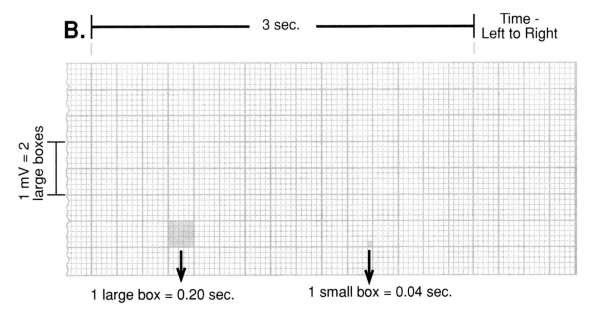

**B.** |——————— 3 sec. ———————|   Time - Left to Right

1 mV = 2 large boxes

1 large box = 0.20 sec.          1 small box = 0.04 sec.

An enlargement of the ECG graph paper showing time and mV.

*Figure 8-1: ECG Graph Paper, a Review*

The isoelectric line is also an important element to be aware of during rhythm analysis. The isoelectric line is not a part of the graph paper, but is important as a reference point. Also called the baseline, the isoelectric line is the marking made on the graph paper by the ECG machine when no electrical current is being detected.

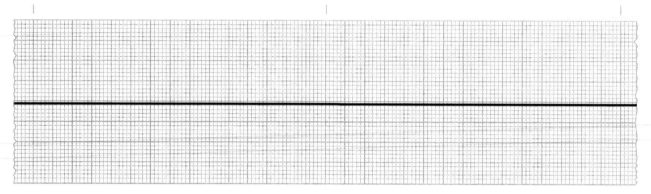

*Figure 8-2: The baseline or isoelectric line is a tracing that occurs when there is no electrical activity being detected by the ECG machine.*

When the heart contracts, electrical current has passed through the heart muscle. The electrical current is recorded as a waveform on the graph paper. As the current is recorded on the paper, the waveform departs from the baseline. A positive waveform is one in which the tracing is recorded above the baseline; and a negative waveform is one in which the tracing is recorded below the baseline. Whether the waveform is positive or negative may be a significant feature in determining the nature of complex rhythms. Waveforms are measured from the point at which they depart from the baseline to the point at which they return to the baseline. The interval between the departure and the return to the baseline is the length of the wave.

## Systematic Rhythm Analysis

The systematic approach to rhythm analysis involves determination of rate, assessment of regularity, and measurement of waveforms. The first step is to determine the heart rate in beats per minute (bpm). The next step is to examine the rhythm to determine if the waveforms occur at regular intervals. The final step is to measure the duration of waveforms: the P wave and the QRS complex. Based on the results of these observations, the rhythm then can be labeled as being NSR (normal sinus rhythm), a variation of NSR, or an abnormal heart rhythm. NSR and its variations are described in this chapter. Abnormal heart rhythms will be discussed in Chapter Nine.

The preliminary step for determining sinus rhythm is to briefly look at the ECG strip. Keep the following in mind: usually, the heart beats at regular intervals. The QRS complex represents the electrical event during the depolarization of the ventricles, and occurs just prior to the mechanical contraction of the ventricle. The QRS complex should appear at regular intervals across the graph paper and should correspond to the patient's pulse rate. Before determining rate and measuring waveforms it is helpful to make some general observations:

- Note if the rhythm seems regular.
- Determine if there is a P wave for every QRS.
- Note if there are extra beats, early beats, or pauses where beats would be expected.

It is important to refrain from coming to any conclusions at this point, and to proceed with the steps in a systematic manner.

The steps involved in ECG analysis allow the technician to fine tune observations and organize them in a way that will lead to an accurate interpretation. The three steps in the interpretation process are explained in detail below.

## 1. Determine Heart Rate

The easiest method for determining the heart rate is to make a quick estimate. This method can be used on both regular and irregular heart rhythms. Remember, the QRS is the electrical impulse which causes the heart to beat. This impulse is what is counted, or measured, to determine the heart rate. The heart beat causes a pulsation that is felt in other parts of the body such as the wrist in the form of a radial pulse. Find the hash marks above the grid on the graph paper. The area between each hash mark represents 3 seconds; one more hash mark out would represent a total of 6 seconds from the starting point. Count the R waves or number of beats during a 6 second period, and then multiply by 10 to get the beats per minute (bpm). For example, if you count 8 QRS complexes during the 6 second period, multiply 8 by 10. The resulting heart rate is 80 bpm.

A more accurate way is to determine how many large squares are between each beat and then memorize what heart rate is associated with each interval. (See Figure 8-4.) However, this method only works on patients with regular rhythms. If the rhythm is irregular, then the overall rate could not be obtained by this method. If this method is used on a patient with an irregular rhythm, it would only apply to the particular interval measured and the overall rate would have to be determined by the method previously described. A heart rate in which one

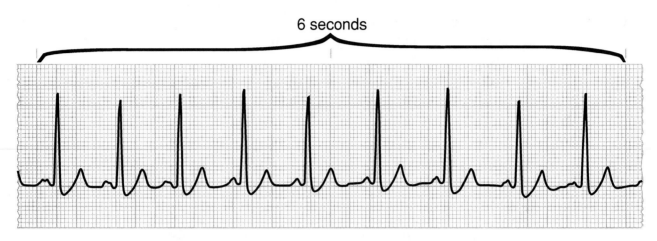

6 seconds

9 beats in 6 sec.
9 X 10 = 90 bpm.

*Figure 8-3: Counting the number of beats that occur in a 6 second interval and multiplying by 10 will provide an approximate number of beats per minute.*

square is between each beat would be a heart rate of 300; two squares, 150 bpm; 3 squares, 100 bpm; 4 squares, 75 bpm; 5 squares, 60 bpm; 6 squares, 50 bpm; 7 squares, 42 bpm; 8 squares, 37 bpm; 9 squares, 21 bpm. Special ECG rulers are available that have the markings and associated heart rates labeled on them to assist in measurement. If the technician is working with electrocardiography everyday, it is best to memorize the rates associated with the interval of squares.

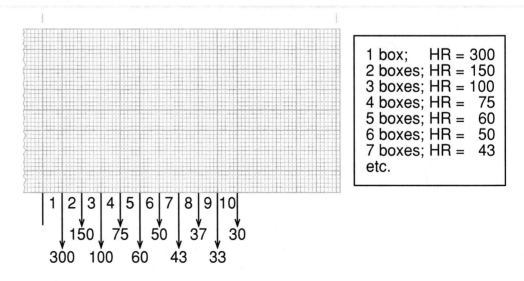

1 box;    HR = 300
2 boxes; HR = 150
3 boxes; HR = 100
4 boxes; HR =  75
5 boxes; HR =  60
6 boxes; HR =  50
7 boxes; HR =  43
etc.

*Figure 8-4: Determining the Heart Rate*

Another method for determining heart rate is mathematical. It should only be used on regular rhythms. The mathematical method is not used often because the square method is easier, but it is helpful to know in that it assists in the understanding of the process and in familiarization with the ECG graph paper.

Count the number of small squares between two beats, or QRS complexes. Then, divide that number into 1500 to get the beats per minute. For example, if you count 20 small squares between QRS complexes, you will divide 1500 by 20 to get a total of 75 bpm. Remember that the horizontal grid represents time; each small square equals 0.04 seconds. Therefore, 1500 small squares comprise one minute. That is why dividing 1500 by the number of small squares between QRSs will give the heart rate during a one minute period.

A similar method for determining heart rate involves counting the large squares. Since each large square represents 0.2 seconds, you need to divide 300 by the number of large squares between QRS complexes. Using the example provided above, 20 small squares would represent the same period of time as 4 large squares from QRS to QRS. By counting the large squares then, the formula would change in this way: 300 ÷ 4 = 75 bpm (the same heart rate as above).

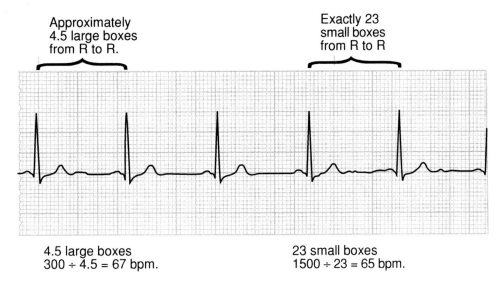

Approximately
4.5 large boxes
from R to R.

Exactly 23
small boxes
from R to R

4.5 large boxes
300 ÷ 4.5 = 67 bpm.

23 small boxes
1500 ÷ 23 = 65 bpm.

*Figure 8-5: Counting the number of large and small boxes in between an R to R interval will provide an approximate number of beats per minute.*

The electrocardiograph, whether it is a 12-Lead electrocardiograph or a cardiac monitor, usually has the capability to determine the heart rate automatically. All new machines will be able to determine the heart rate, display it on the monitor, and print it on the graph paper; but older machines may not have the capability to determine the heart rate. Even if the equipment being used can determine the rate, it is still important for whoever is analyzing the rhythm to be able to determine the heart rate independently and check it against the heart rate determined by the heart monitor. It is important to know that the determination of the heart rate is correct because a significant part of the analysis rests on the heart rate.

## 2. Determine if Rhythm is Regular or Irregular

Briefly examine the rhythm strip and note any obvious irregularities. There may be a grouping of beats, gaps, or pauses, or it may seem that the QRSs appear at regular intervals. After this brief examination of the rhythm you should have an idea of whether the rhythm is regular or irregular. Now you have to confirm your initial impression by actually measuring the distance between the QRS complexes.

There are several ways of measuring the distance between QRSs. The first step is to locate the tall pointed portion of the QRS. When the complex is mostly positive (above the baseline), the R wave is the tallest part of the QRS. However, since the R wave is considered to be a positive waveform, if the main part of the QRS deflection is negative (below the baseline), then the pointed part of the complex is the S wave, or in some cases referred to as the QS wave. (See Figure 8-10 D, later in this chapter.) Whether the complex is positive or negative depends on what lead the monitor is recording, and also on the patient's underlying disease and/or if there are any conduction abnormalities. At this point it doesn't matter if you are dealing with a positive or negative QRS. But what IS important is to locate the large, pointed part of the QRS and be able to identify it consistently.

One method of determining the interval is to count the squares, small or large, between two QRS complexes. The number of squares should be the same between each complex in order to conclude that the rhythm is regular. Of course, the number of squares between complexes may be difficult to measure because it will be hard to find an R wave or S wave that occurs directly on a line. Also, there most likely will not be an exact whole number of squares, but rather a whole number of squares and a fraction of a square. When starting out in ECG interpretation, the process of counting squares may make the activity more meaningful. It is more important to remember the reason why you are doing an activity rather than just coming up with a number. The time interval that occurs between QRS complexes should be the same in order for the rhythm to be determined as regular. There are, however, easier ways to determine the regularity of a heart rhythm than counting squares.

One of the easier methods for assessing regularity involves using a blank piece of paper and a pencil or pen. Place the blank paper over the ECG strip so that only the tips of the QRS complexes are visible. Mark the blank paper where each tip (See Figure 8-6) occurs. The usual procedure is to mark three QRS spikes. Be careful not to move the paper while marking the spikes. Now, move the paper down to the second QRS that was marked; place the first mark on the second complex and check to see if the rest of the marks match up with a QRS spike. Move the paper down to the next complex and repeat the procedure. If the QRS complexes occur at regular intervals, then the marks on the paper will consistently match up with the QRS complexes. This process is called "marching out the QRSs." If the rhythm is determined to be regular, another way to describe this is to say the R waves, or QRS complexes, "march out."

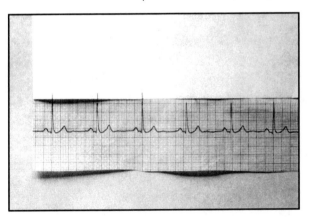

**A.** Place a blank piece of paper at the tips of the R wave and mark out two cycles of R to R intervals by making a mark that corresponds to each of the first three R waves on the blank paper.

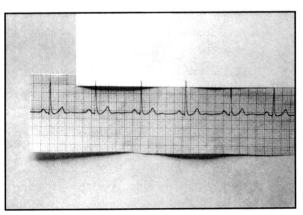

**B.** Move the paper down one cycle by placing the first mark over the second R wave. If the second and third marks fall on R waves, the rhythm is regular (the R to R intervals are the same for these beats). Continue to move the paper down one cycle until the whole strip has been examined for regularity.

*Figure 8-6: A Paper and Pencil Method for Determining Regularity*

**calipers:**
a metal tool used to assist in the accurate measurement of waveforms.

Another method for determining regularity is by using **calipers**. Most professionals who frequently work with ECGs and heart rhythm recordings use calipers as their primary tool. Calipers look a little like a protractor. (See Figure 8-7.) The tool consists of two arms, each with sharp, pointed tips at one end. The arms are connected at the unpointed ends by a pivot joint. The pointed ends can be moved away from each other to a

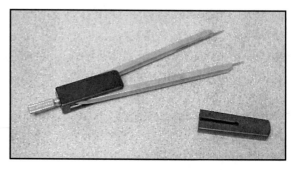

Figure 8-7: Calipers are used to measure waveforms and determine their regularity on the ECG.

certain length, and the tension can be adjusted so that the distance between the pointed tips will not slip during the measurement process. There usually is a screw at the pivot end that adjusts the tension. The screw should be adjusted so that the arms can move with some pressure, but will not slip with the light pressure of holding the device in one hand.

To use the calipers, place one point on the QRS complex, either at the peak of the spike or at the beginning of the QRS complex. Place the point of the other arm at the same point on the next QRS complex and adjust the tension of the caliper so the distance between these points is locked. Pivot the caliper on the arm that is placed on the second QRS in a way that turns the caliper in a half circle and moves the arm off of the first complex and onto the third complex. The arm should fall on the same place on the third complex as it left on the first complex. If the interval doesn't match, then note if it falls short or beyond the third complex. If the interval matches, then continue pivoting until the whole strip is evaluated. If irregularities are noted, then you may want to reset the caliper to an interval that appears in the middle of the ECG strip in order to see if there are any regular intervals on the strip. This process may seem confusing at first because there is a large range of variation. A heart rhythm strip may appear regular and yet, when measured, may have slight irregularities. A rhythm strip may have irregularities at the beginning of the strip, and then become regular in the middle or toward the end of the strip. So, it is important to examine the WHOLE strip and to note any irregularities. Analysis of the entire strip may help in the final interpretation of the ECG.

At the end of analysis, you should be able to say that the rhythm is **regular**, **irregular**, or **irregularly irregular**. Regular means that the QRS occurs at regular intervals. Irregular can mean two things: it can mean a patterned irregularity (eg, every third beat is early), or random irregularity without a pattern (irregularly irregular). Irregular is the broad term for both patterned and nonpatterned irregularities. Sometimes it is helpful to note a pattern or to note that the irregular beats occur without a pattern; they are irregularly irregular.

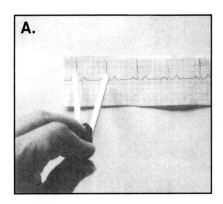 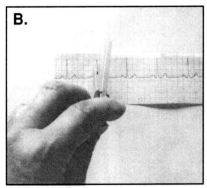 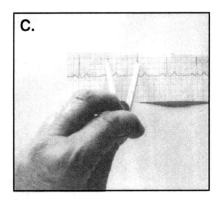

A. Adjust the calipers so that the points are in contact with the R waves of the first two QRS complexes.
B. Pivot the calipers so that the first point lifts up and the second point remains in contact with the second R wave.
C. Allow the first point to make a half circle and land on the paper. If the rhythm is regular as in the picture, the point will land directly on the third R wave. Continue to pivot the calipers in half circles until the entire strip is measured and examined for regularity.

*Figure 8-8: Using Calipers to Determine Regularity*

## 3. Measure Waveforms

Before beginning a discussion of the measurement of waveforms, a quick review of the waveforms may be helpful. The baseline, or isoelectric line, is the straight line that indicates there is no perceptible electrical activity occurring. Waveforms are measured in reference to the baseline. The heart is at rest, or in diastole, during the period of time when the waveform is flat and at baseline.

The P wave is the first wave to occur. The P wave represents the travel of electrical current through the atria. Since the atria are small, the P wave is small and rounded, and the current travels relatively slowly through the atria. The P wave may be positive or negative, depending on the lead. Then, the electrical current reaches the ventricles. The ventricles are larger than the atria and the electrical current travels relatively quickly through the ventricles (because of the bundle branches and the Purkinje fibers). The passage of electrical current through the ventricle gives the QRS complex its characteristics of being tall and spiky, and short in duration when compared to the P wave. The QRS complex may be positive or negative, depending on the lead. After the QRS occurs the small, rounded T wave appears, which represents the repolarization of the ventricles. Finally, the T wave returns to baseline and the cycle begins again, within the atria.

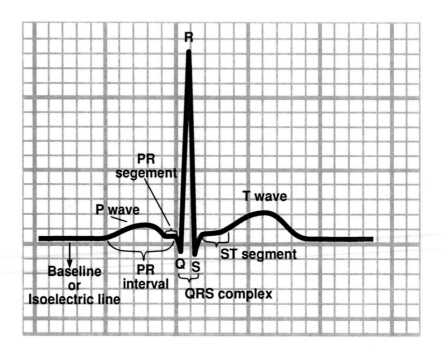

*Figure 8-9: The Components of the ECG Waveform*

Remember, in order for the sinus mechanism (the origin of the heart beat in the SA node) to be assessed as operational, there should be a P wave for every QRS. The electrical current starts in the right atria in the sinoatrial node (SA node), and travels down to the ventricles. If there is no P wave detected, then the electrical impulse is originating in another part of the heart, not in the SA node. In cases like this, the heart rhythm cannot be classified as normal sinus rhythm (NSR).

The easiest way to measure waveforms is by using the calipers. Place the tip of one caliper arm at the beginning of the wave to be measured and place the other tip at the end of the wave. The beginning of the waveform is usually when the wave begins to move away from the baseline. The end of the wave is identified either when it returns to baseline or when the beginning of another wave is noted. Because the beginning of a wave will most likely NOT coincide with the beginning of a square on the graph paper, the use of a caliper will assist in accurate measurement. Once the interval of the wave is captured between the points of the caliper, move the caliper to another part of the graph paper and put one point at the beginning of a large square, then count how many small or large squares fall within the caliper points. When moving the caliper be careful not to move the distance between the tips (this is the length of the measured wave). Remember that waveforms are measured in seconds, and each small square equals 0.04 seconds and each large square equals 0.20 seconds. So, if a waveform is 3 small squares, then the duration of the wave is 0.12 seconds (3 x 0.04 = 0.12). If a waveform is 4 small squares, then the duration of the wave is 0.16 seconds (4 x 0.04 = 0.16). If a waveform is 5 small squares, that is the same as 1 large square, then the duration of the wave is 0.20 seconds (5 x 0.04 = 0.20). If a waveform is 3.5 small squares, then the duration of the wave is 0.14 seconds.

- **PR interval** – Measure the P wave from the beginning of the P wave (the point at which the wave departs from the baseline) to the beginning of the QRS complex. The end of the P wave is considered to be at the beginning of the QRS complex. The P wave may or may not return to baseline before the start of the QRS. You will be able to tell when the QRS has started because of its sharp angles and points when compared to the gently rounded P wave. This interval should measure from 0.12 to 0.20 seconds, or from 3 small squares to one large square. If the PR interval measures within these limits, then it can be established that the SA node is functioning properly.

- **QRS complex** – Begin measuring the QRS complex at the start of the first small, sharp deflection after the P wave, and end the measurement when the wave returns to baseline or at the start of the T wave. The initial spike is called the Q wave. In Lead I it would be negative, then the R wave will spike upwards in a tall wave. Finally, the S wave will be a small negative deflection, with a possible return to baseline. However, the S wave may not return to baseline before the beginning of the T wave. This may make it difficult to determine the end of the QRS, but after some practice, the end of the QRS will become apparent. In $V_1$ there really is no Q wave. There is only a tiny R wave, a large negative S wave, and then a return to baseline. Each lead used has a slightly different configuration for the QRS. For a beginning student in ECG rhythm analysis it is important to focus on identifying the sharp deflections, whether positive or negative, as the QRS complex and to know that there are many variations in its appearance, depending on the lead used and the patient's underlying physiology and disease process. A patient who has a **heart block** may have several large positive and negative spikes that make up one QRS complex. Whether or not all the components are visible, the waveform that follows the P wave is the depolarization of the ventricles and is most often referred to as the QRS, or sometimes the R wave (if there is one main positive deflection). This may be confusing at first, but after working with ECGs and rhythm analysis for a time it will become easier. The duration of the QRS complex should measure from 0.04 seconds to 0.10 seconds. That means the waveform should not be shorter than 1 small square and should not be longer than about 2.5 small squares.

**heart block:** a disturbance in the conduction system of the heart.

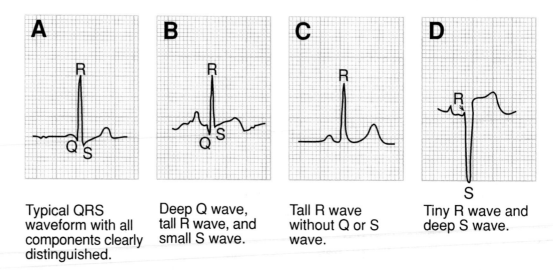

| **A** | **B** | **C** | **D** |
|---|---|---|---|
| Typical QRS waveform with all components clearly distinguished. | Deep Q wave, tall R wave, and small S wave. | Tall R wave without Q or S wave. | Tiny R wave and deep S wave. |

Each of these waveforms is called a QRS—even if all components are not present—because the "QRS" represents ventricular depolarization. The exact configuration depends on the lead used and the patient's condition. Remember to start the measurement when the wave departs from the baseline and end the measurement when the wave returns to the baseline or levels off.

*Figure 8-10: Variations of QRS*

- **ST segment** – The ST segment, the portion of the T wave that connects to the QRS complex, is not routinely used in rhythm analysis. The ST segment is normally flat. But, injury to the heart wall, myocardial infarction, or myocardial ischemia may cause the ST segment on a 12-Lead ECG to be elevated (above the baseline) or even depressed (below the baseline). Certain abnormal rhythms may also have an ST segment that does not return to baseline. This segment is not measured, but is noted to be elevated or at baseline.

- **T wave** – The T wave is not usually measured and is not part of the criteria used in rhythm analysis. The importance of the T wave is its usefulness in determining if ischemia is present. The T wave may be inverted (flipped upside down) if coronary artery disease and ischemia are present. This wave is only used in advanced 12-Lead ECG analysis.

- **QT interval** – The QT interval usually is not used in basic rhythm analysis. If it is used, it is measured from the beginning of the QRS to the end of the T wave (where the T wave returns to baseline). There is no set interval duration for the QT interval because it varies with the heart rate and depends on the sex of the patient. As a rule of thumb, the QT interval should not be more that half of the R to R interval. Special tables and formulas are used to derive the QT interval, based on the heart rate.

# Rhythm Interpretation

The heart rhythms discussed in this chapter include **normal sinus rhythm (NSR)** and variations of normal sinus rhythm. Since these rhythms are considered "normal," patients experiencing these rhythms may not require treatment unless they have additional symptoms or complications, such as fatigue, light-headedness, or pain.

The criteria for all heart rhythms in this chapter and the next will follow the same format. The criteria for the rate, the regularity, and the waveform will be listed below the name of the heart rhythm. This listing will be followed by a brief explanation of the heart rhythm and an illustration.

The following are descriptions of normal sinus rhythm and variations of normal sinus rhythm.

## Normal Sinus Rhythm

**Heart rate:** 60 – 100 bpm.

**Regularity of R to R interval:** Regular.

**Waveforms:** There is a P wave for every QRS.

- **PR interval:** 0.12 – 0.20 seconds.
- **QRS:** 0.04 – 0.10 seconds.

Normal sinus rhythm (NSR) is the regular rhythm that is produced by the electrical impulse originating in the SA node, which travels to the ventricles via the bundle branches, and results in the coordinated contraction of the atria and ventricles. The terms *regular sinus rhythm* or *sinus rhythm* are used interchangeably with NSR. This book will use the term *NSR*, but other terms may also be used.

**normal sinus rhythm (NSR)** or **regular sinus rhythm (RSR):** a heart rhythm that originates in the sinus node and travels down the normal route of the conduction system to the cardiac muscle , resulting in contraction of the heart muscle. On graph paper the rhythm is regular (the beats occur evenly), and the P wave, QRS, and T wave have usual appearances and measurements. The rate is between 60-100 beats per minute.

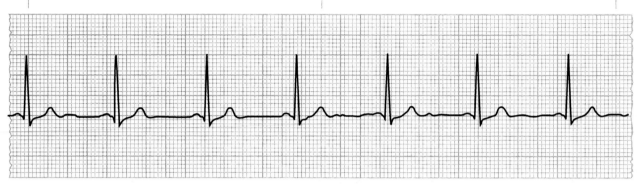

Examine the strip. Note that there is a P wave for every QRS. Also note that it appears regular. Measure with calipers to confirm regularity. Estimate the rate by counting the complexes in the 6 second bracket. There are six complexes, so multiply that by 10 to get 60 beats per minute. For a more precise heart rate, use the calipers to determine how many large boxes are between one R to R interval. The R to R interval encompasses more than four large boxes, but less than five; so the heart rate is about 64 bpm.

**Summary**

**Rate** = 64 bpm. Regular rhythm. P wave for every QRS. **PR interval** = 0.12 sec. **QRS** = 0.08 sec. Criteria for NSR met.

*Figure 8-11: Normal Sinus Rhythm (NSR)*

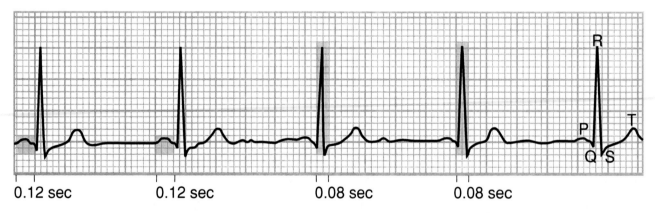

0.12 sec          0.12 sec          0.08 sec          0.08 sec

The strip in Figure 8-11 is enlarged in order to distinguish the waveforms more easily. In the first two complexes the P wave is highlighted to show that 3 small boxes (0.12 sec.) is the duration of the P wave. In the third and fourth complex the QRS is highlighted to demonstrate that the QRS duration is 0.08 sec.

*Figure 8-12: NSR – Enlarged*

## Sinus Bradycardia

**Heart rate:** Below 60 bpm.

**Regularity of R to R interval:** Regular.

**Waveforms:** One P wave for each QRS.

- **PR interval:** 0.12 – 0.20 seconds.
- **QRS:** 0.04 – 0.10 seconds.

**Sinus bradycardia** refers to a heart rhythm that is slower than 60 bpm. All other criteria are the same as for NSR. It may be normal for many people to have a resting heart rate in the 50 bpm range, especially if they are athletes. Someone who is in good physical condition, like an athlete, will have a slower heart rate. This is because physical conditioning causes the heart to beat more efficiently, resulting in a slower heart rate. Similarly, a person's heart rate may drop to 50 bpm or slower when he or she is asleep. The heart rate drops because the body's needs are minimal while asleep, so the heart doesn't need to beat as fast. Therefore, sinus bradycardia does not necessarily mean that pathology is present; it may be a normal variation. Most people can tolerate a bradycardia that is as slow as 50 bpm and maybe even as slow as 40 bpm. However, many people will begin to experience ill effects from a heart rate of 40 bpm and below.

When evaluating a rhythm disturbance or a rhythm variation, it is important to consider the patient and how he or she responds to the rhythm. If the patient is having symptoms with the lower heart rate, then this may not be a patient's norm, and may indicate a disease process. Symptoms may include light-headedness, dizziness, or syncope (fainting). The patient's medications should also be considered. Medications used to treat heart disease may cause the heartbeat to slow down. It may be that the patient's dosage of medication may be too high, causing the heart rate to become dangerously slow. In this case, the patient's bradycardia should be called to the attention of the physician or nurse, so that adjustments to the medication dosage can be made.

**sinus bradycardia:** a heart rhythm that originates in the SA node. The rhythm is regular and all waveforms have normal morphology (shape) and duration, but the heart rate is less than 60 bpm.

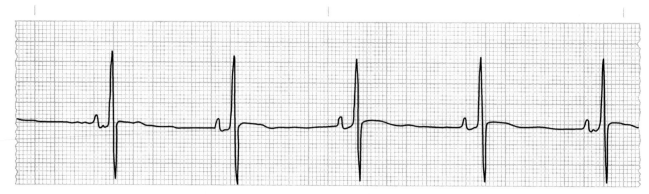

**Heart Rate (HR):** 5 complexes in a 6 second period.
   5 X 10 = 50 bpm.
   R to R interval measures slightly more than 6 large boxes, which is about 49 bpm.
**Regularity of R to R interval:** Regular
**Waveforms:** P wave for every QRS
   **PR interval:** 0.14 sec.
   **QRS:** 0.10 sec

*Figure 8-13: Sinus Bradycardia*

## Sinus Tachycardia

**Heart rate:** 100 – 180 bpm.

**Regularity of R to R interval:** Regular, unless gradually accelerating (getting faster) or decelerating (slowing).

**Waveforms:** One P wave for every QRS.

- **PR interval:** 0.12 – 0.20 seconds (may shorten slightly with rapid rate).

- **QRS:** 0.04 – 0.10 seconds.

**sinus tachycardia:** a heart rhythm that originates in the SA node. The rhythm is regular and all waveforms have normal morphology and duration, but the heart rate is more than 100 bpm.

**Sinus tachycardia** occurs when the patient's heart rate is greater than 100 bpm. During exercise, the heart rate can safely go above 180 bpm. However, the rate of the SA node does not usually conduct impulses greater than 180 bpm. Sinus tachycardia usually signals a physiologic response to a physical need or condition. If a person is exercising, the body will require an increase in oxygen and nutrients. This increased need is the reason for the rise in the heart rate during exercise. This is normal and desirable. If someone exercises and the heart rate does not increase, then the body will not be able to sustain the exercise. Sinus tachycardia may also indicate a disease or condition such as anxiety, fever, pain, infection, drug effects, hemorrhage, or hormone imbalance. The underlying disease condition usually needs to be addressed in order to cure the tachycardia.

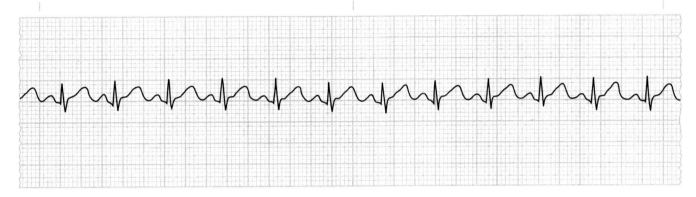

**HR:** 12 complexes in a 6 second period.
    12 X 10 = 120 bpm.
    R to R duration: 2 ¹/₂ large boxes = 125 bpm.
**Regularity of R to R interval:** Regular
**Waveforms:** P wave for every QRS
  **PR interval:** 0.16 seconds
  **QRS:** 0.08 seconds

*Figure 8-14: Sinus Tachycardia*

## Sinus Arrhythmia

**Heart rate:** 60-100 bpm.

**Regularity of R to R interval:** Irregular, the rhythm changes with the respiratory cycle. It will gradually speed up with inspiration and gradually slow down with exhalation.

**Waveforms:** There is a P wave for each QRS.

- **PR interval:** 0.12 – 0.20 seconds.

- **QRS:** 0.04 – 0.10 seconds.

**Sinus arrhythmia** is also a variation of sinus rhythm (NSR). It occurs very gradually, and it may be imperceptible at first. The speeding of the rate occurs gradually with inhalation (taking a breath into the lungs); the slowing of the rate occurs gradually with exhalation (releasing air from the lungs). This occurs gradually and cyclically with the respiratory (breathing) cycle. This rhythm is not clinically significant to a patient's condition. As an ECG technician you need to be aware that it can occur, but it will not affect the diagnosis.

**sinus arrhythmia:** variation of normal sinus rhythm in which the rhythm is initiated from the sinus node and meets all criteria for NSR except that it is irregular. The rhythm varies with respiration, speeding up with inspiration and slowing with expiration.

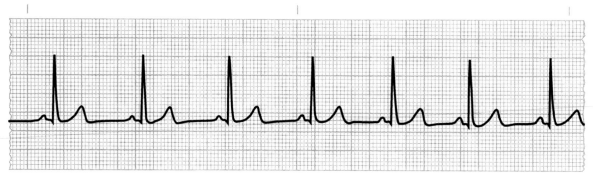

**HR:** The overall rate is an average of 70 bpm. (7 complexes during the 6 second interval; 7 X 10 = 70.)

**Regularity of R to R interval:** Irregular, the R to R interval gradually shortens. The longest R to R is between the first two beats and measures almost 5 large boxes (about 64 bpm). The shortest R to R is between beats 5 and 6 and measures a little more than 4 large boxes (about 74 bpm). So the rate ranges from 64 to 74, or between four and five large boxes.

**Waveforms:**

    **PR interval:** 0.14 seconds.

    **QRS:** 0.08 seconds.

Since it is a gradual shortening and lengthening of the R to R interval (it begins to lengthen again after beat 6), then this probably demonstrates a sinus arrhythmia. You may have to look at a longer tracing to see the cyclical shortening and lengthening of the R to R interval.

Sinus arrhythmia is a normal variation that occurs with respiration. It is not clinically significant.

*Figure 8-15: Sinus Arrhythmia*

# Chapter Summary

ECG graph paper is divided into boxes which measure time. These boxes are used to determine heart rate and the length of the waveforms. Normal sinus rhythm is a heart beat that originates in the SA node, travels down the atria to the AV node, and moves to the ventricles via the bundle branches. NSR is present with these parameters: heart rate = 60 to 100 bpm; PR interval = 0.12 to 0.20; QRS = 0.04 to 0.10 seconds; and the R to R interval is regular. Normal variations include sinus bradycardia, sinus tachycardia, and sinus arrhythmia.

Name_____

Date_____

# Student Enrichment Activities

**Analyze the rhythm strips below. Determine the rate and regularity of the waveforms, and then measure them. Note any variations from NSR and label the strips with an interpretation.**

1. • Rate _____     • QRS _____

   • Regularity _____         • Abnormal beats _____

   • PR interval _____          • Interpretation _____

2. • Rate _____     • QRS _____

   • Regularity _____         • Abnormal beats _____

   • PR interval _____          • Interpretation _____

**3.**
- Rate _____
- Regularity _____
- PR interval _____
- QRS _____
- Abnormal beats _____
- Interpretation _____

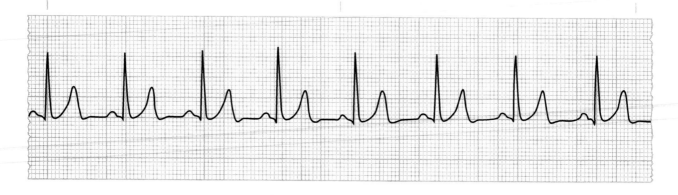

**4.**
- Rate _____
- Regularity _____
- PR interval _____
- QRS _____
- Abnormal beats _____
- Interpretation _____

Name_____

Date_____

5.  • Rate _____        • QRS _____

    • Regularity _____        • Abnormal beats _____

    • PR interval _____        • Interpretation _____

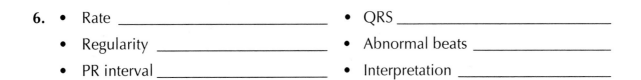

6.  • Rate _____        • QRS _____

    • Regularity _____        • Abnormal beats _____

    • PR interval _____        • Interpretation _____

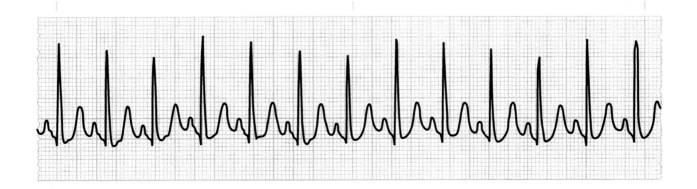

7. • Rate _____     • QRS _____

   • Regularity _____     • Abnormal beats _____

   • PR interval _____     • Interpretation _____

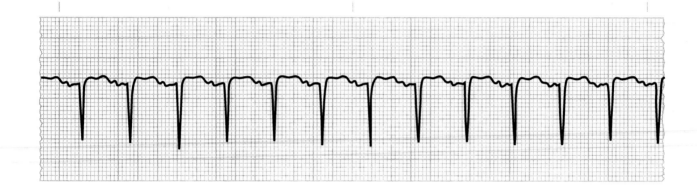

8. • Rate _____     • QRS _____

   • Regularity _____     • Abnormal beats _____

   • PR interval _____     • Interpretation _____

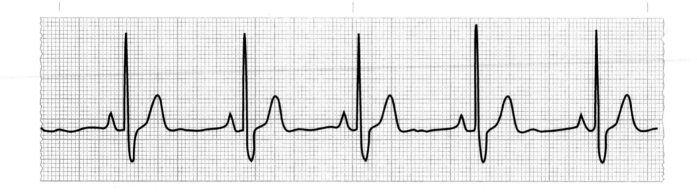

Name_____

Date_____

9. • Rate _____        • QRS _____

   • Regularity _____        • Abnormal beats _____

   • PR interval _____        • Interpretation _____

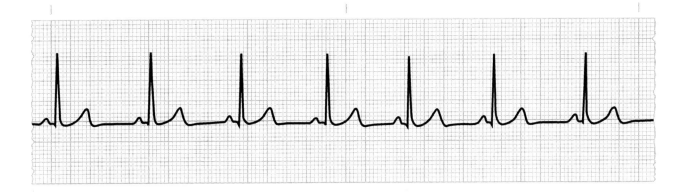

**Circle the letter of the best answer.**

10. Sinus bradycardia occurs when the heart rate is

    A. less than 40

    B. 40 – 80

    C. less than 60

    D. 60 – 100

11. Sinus tachycardia occurs when the heart rate is

    A. 60 – 100

    B. 100 –180

    C. less than 90

    D. greater than 60

12. The rate of NSR is

    A. 60 – 120

    B. 50 – 100

    C. greater than 60

    D. 60 – 100

**Complete the following statements.**

13. _____ _____ is a normal variation of NSR that occurs when the heart rate varies with respiration.

14. _____ _____ is a normal variation of NSR that may occur when the patient is anxious, in pain, or has a fever.

15. _____ _____ is a normal variation of NSR that may occur in athletes or when the patient is asleep.

16. In NSR the PR interval usually measures _____ to _____ seconds or _____ to _____ small squares.

17. In NSR the QRS measures _____ to _____ seconds or about _____ to _____small squares.

18. In NSR every P wave is followed by a _____.

19. Twelve small squares on the ECG graph paper equals _____ seconds.

20. Five large squares on the ECG graph paper equals _____ seconds.

21. To determine the heart rate, measure the _____ to _____ interval and determine the number of small squares in this interval; then divide that number into 1500.

22. If there are 20 small squares between QRS complexes, what is the heart rate? _____

Name_____

Date_____


**23.** If there are 30 small squares between QRS complexes what is the heart rate?

_____


**24.** Ten small squares equal _____ large squares on the ECG graph paper.


**25.** _____ large squares on the ECG graph paper equal one minute.


**26.** If there are four large squares between QRS complexes, then the heart rate is

_____.


**27.** If there are two large squares between QRS complexes, then the heart rate is

_____.


**28.** If there are five large squares between QRS complexes, then the heart rate is

_____.


**29.** If the heart rate is irregular, the heart rate may be determined by _____ the number of _____ complexes within _____ seconds and multiplying by _____.


**30.** The hash marks above the grid at the top of the ECG paper occur every

_____ seconds.

8-28

# Chapter Nine
# Analysis and Identification of Abnormal Heart Rhythms

## *Objectives*

After completing this chapter, you should be able to
do the following:

1. Define and correctly spell each of the key terms.

2. Name three abnormal heart rhythms that originate in the atria of the heart.

3. Name three abnormal heart rhythms that originate in the ventricles of the heart.

4. Name three abnormal heart rhythms that occur because of abnormalities that block the conduction system of the heart.

5. Name three heart rhythms that indicate a medical emergency.

# Key Terms

- asystole
- atrial fibrillation
- atrial flutter
- bundle branch block (BBB)
- first degree AV heart block
- idioventricular rhythm
- junctional escape
- pacemaker rhythm
- paroxysmal atrial tachycardia (PAT)
- premature atrial contraction (PAC)
- premature junctional contraction (PJC)
- premature ventricular contraction (PVC)
- second degree AV heart block: Mobitz Type I
- second degree AV heart block: Mobitz Type II
- supraventricular tachycardia (SVT)
- third degree AV heart block
- ventricular fibrillation
- ventricular tachycardia (VT)

# Introduction

Abnormal heartbeats can originate in the atria or the ventricles as a result of damage or chemical imbalance. Abnormal heart beats can occur as isolated incidences or they can be continuous and last over long periods of time. When they occur in an isolated instance, treatment may not be indicated. However, if the abnormal rhythm is continuous, prompt treatment and emergency measures may be required.

# Atrial Arrhythmias

Atrial arrhythmias cause the heart to beat irregularly. They are called atrial arrhythmias because the electrical impulses that cause the extra heart beats originate in the atria instead of in the sinoatrial node (SA node). Remember that the SA node is specialized conduction tissue located in the high right atrium. Atrial arrhythmias, therefore, originate in other parts of the right atrium or in the left atrium. These arrhythmias can be mild rhythm disturbances that may be accompanied by minimal symptoms; or, in some cases, a patient may experience no symptoms at all. In extreme cases, these rhythm disturbances can cause serious health problems that are accompanied by severe symptoms.

It is important to study ECG strips in a systematic manner. Always examine the strip with the same method, step by step, so that no feature will be overlooked or misinterpreted. Determine the heart rate, assess the regularity of the beat, and measure the waveforms. Notice any unusual features and determine if each P wave is followed by a QRS.

## Premature Atrial Contraction (PAC)

**Rate:** 60 – 100 bpm.

**Regularity:** Irregular or irregularly irregular. The premature beat will come in earlier than expected.

**Waveforms:** There is a P wave for each QRS, but the P wave of the premature beat may have a different morphology (form).

- **PR interval:** 0.12 – 0.20 seconds.

- **QRS:** 0.04 – 0.10 seconds.

The **premature atrial contraction**, or PAC, is caused by an electrical impulse that originates in the atria, outside of the SA node. It is called premature because it fires before the natural, dominant pacemaker (the SA node) has a chance to produce an impulse. This early impulse may be caused by "irritability" in the atria. The irritability, which is a physiologic dysfunction, may be the result of several conditions, including electrolyte imbalance, CAD, or valvular disease. When examining a rhythm strip with PACs it will be evident that the intervals are irregular; the PAC comes in earlier than a sinus beat (a beat generated by the SA node). This irregularity can be noted during a brief overview of the strip or when measuring for rate and regularity. The early complex will look fairly normal except for the fact that it is early. The P wave may have a different shape and look slightly different because it is coming from a different area in the atria, outside of the dominant pacemaker. The P wave may also be difficult to locate because it may be distorted; if it occurs close to the end of the T wave of the previous normal beat, it may blend into the T wave. This distorts the P wave and in a PAC makes it hard to locate. A P wave will definitely be present, but it may be difficult to find. The QRS will be normal. Notice that after the PAC occurs, the SA node "resets" itself. This is because the SA node has set the heart rate based on the PAC rather than from the last normal beat.

**premature atrial contraction (PAC):** an early heart beat that originates in the atria outside of the SA node as a result of atrial irritability.

The PACs may occur infrequently or frequently. If they occur frequently, they may appear in a pattern (eg, every other beat, or every third beat). The recurring pattern is called **atrial bigeminy** if it occurs every other beat, and **atrial trigeminy** if it occurs every third beat. Unless they occur frequently, the patient usually will not notice PACs. *Infrequent* is a relative term; it can be used to refer to PACs that occur once per minute to once per hour. *Frequent* is also a relative term; it usually refers to more than six occurrences per minute.

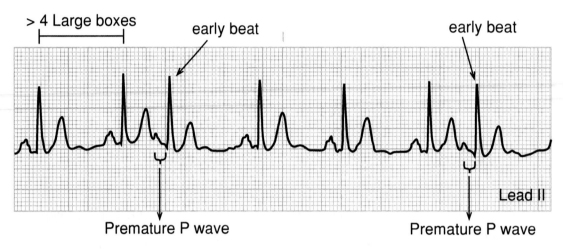

**Rate:** The heart rate of the regular beats is about 70 bpm. Between beats 1 and 2, and between beats 4 and 5, and 5 and 6, the R to R interval is constant at a little more than 4 boxes, which equals 70 bpm.

**Regularity:** Irregular. Beats 3 and 7 are early, or premature.

**Waveforms:** P wave for every QRS.

    **PR:** 0.20 seconds on normal beats.

    **QRS:** 0.08 seconds

P wave of early beat upright.

QRS of early beat narrow and the same as sinus beat.

Interpretation: NSR with PACs

*Figure 9-1: Premature Atrial Contraction (PAC)*

## Paroxysmal Atrial Tachycardia

    **Rate:** 160 – 220 bpm.

    **Regularity:** Regular.

    **Waveforms:** The P wave may be buried in the T wave at a very fast rate and may be difficult to distinguish.

        • **PR interval:** 0.12 – 0.20 seconds.

        • **QRS:** 0.04 – 0.10 seconds.

**Paroxysmal atrial tachycardia** (PAT) is a rapid burst of tachycardia that comes from an area of the atrium outside of the SA node. *Paroxysmal* means that the tachycardia starts and stops suddenly. This type of tachycardia is caused by an irritable or damaged part of the atria that fires rapidly and repeatedly. The increased rate usually lasts only a few seconds and slows to a normal sinus rhythm spontaneously. In order to be classified as an atrial tachycardia, P waves must be present; but again, it may be difficult to distinguish them from the T waves. This is because the rate is so rapid that the P waves occur at the end of the T waves and may be buried inside of those waves. To determine whether a P wave is present within the T wave, compare the T wave of the tachycardia to the T wave of a normal beat. If there is an extra bump in the T wave of the abnormal beat, then the bump most likely represents a P wave. The QRS complex will be normal.

**paroxysmal atrial tachycardia:** a rapid burst of tachycardia that comes from an area of the atrium outside of the SA node with present but often difficult to distinguish P waves.

A patient with PAT may experience symptoms that are minor, such as a fluttering in the chest. Or, the patient may experience more severe symptoms such as chest pain, shortness of breath, or dizziness.

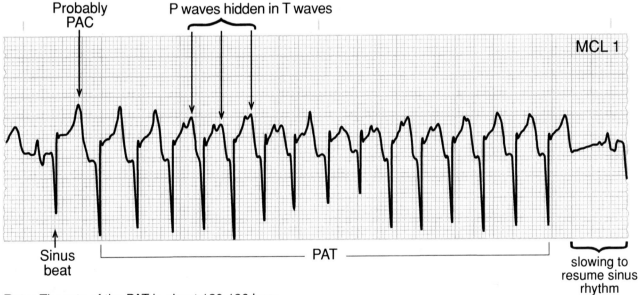

**Rate:** The rate of the PAT is about 180-190 bpm.
**Regularity:** Beginning of PAT is slightly irregular, then it becomes more regular. PAT starts and stops suddenly. It is probably initiated by PAC.
**Waveforms:**
    **PR:** 0.16 seconds in sinus beat.
    **QRS:** 0.06 seconds in sinus beats and PAT.
The underlying rhythm is NSR. The rapid rhythm that starts and stops suddenly is PAT because P waves are hidden in the T waves and the QRS is narrower or the same as in NSR.

*Figure 9-2: Paroxysmal Atrial Tachycardia (PAT)*

## Atrial Flutter

**Rate:** The ventricular rate will be variable to a rate of 150 - 170 bpm.

**Regularity:** Regular or irregular.

**Waveforms:** Flutter waves instead of P waves, the QRS will be normal.

- **PR interval:** None present. Flutter waves appear in a regular sawtooth form at a rate of 250 - 350 per minute.

- **QRS:** 0.04 – 0.10 seconds.

**atrial flutter:** a heart rhythm that originates from the same location in the atria, resulting in atrial activity that creates a characteristic sawtooth waveform that is very fast. Some of the atrial impulses are transmitted to the ventricles resulting in a fast QRS and ventricular contraction. The QRS may be regular or irregular.

**Atrial flutter** has characteristic flutter waves that appear in a regular sawtooth form. Each flutter wave is jagged and triangular, and occurs regularly at a rate of about 300 per minute. The flutter originates from one location in the atria outside of the SA node. The atrioventricular (AV) node, at the bottom of the right atrium, protects the ventricle from beating too fast. It will not conduct all of the flutter waves to the ventricle, but will filter some out. This prevents the ventricle from being overwhelmed with activity. If all of the flutter waves were conducted, it would cause ventricular standstill or collapse because the ventricle is not capable of pumping that fast. So, the ventricular rate will be slower than the flutter rate. The ventricular rate is variable and depends on the level of block; it can reach 150 - 170 bpm. The QRS may appear following every other flutter wave, following every third, following every fourth, or less frequently. If ventricular conduction occurs following every other flutter wave, it is called atrial flutter with 2:1 block. If it occurs following every third flutter wave, it is said to be an atrial flutter with a 3:1 block. If it occurs following every fourth flutter wave, it is said to be an atrial flutter with a 4:1 block, and so on.

Consider these patterns when determining the degree of block. The conduction may also be variable, meaning that the AV node doesn't conduct at a fixed ratio. For example, it may conduct after three flutter waves, then after five flutter waves, and then after two flutter waves, etc. This is called *atrial flutter with variable ventricular response*. So it is evident that atrial flutter can be very regular or irregular. The flutter waves from the atria are regular, but they may be hard to detect because a flutter wave may be hiding in the QRS.

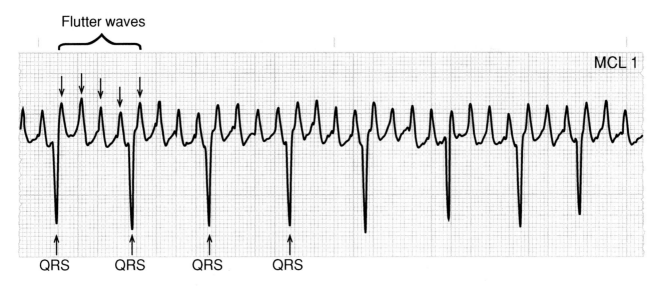

**Rate:** Ventricular rate, about 80 bpm.

**Regularity:** First part of strip QRSs are regular, the second half are irregular.

**Waveforms:**

    **PR:** None. Flutter waves are present throughout the strip. Flutter waves occur regularly at a rate of 300 per minute (1 box). The presence of the classic "sawtooth" morphology of the flutter waves indicates that this is atrial flutter.

    **QRS:** Measures 0.06 second and occurs at a variable rate of approximately 80 bpm.

*Figure 9-3: Atrial Flutter*

## Atrial Fibrillation

**Rate:** 100 – 180 bpm.

**Regularity:** Irregularly irregular.

**Waveforms:** Atrial activity is chaotic and QRS morphology will appear normal.

- **PR interval:** No P wave present.
- **QRS:** 0.04 – 0.10 seconds.

There is no organized contraction of the atria in **atrial fibrillation**. The source of the electrical impulse originates in multiple locations within the atria at the same time. The impulses fire rapidly and chaotically, so the atrial muscle gets multiple messages to contract. The disorganization caused by this condition results in the atria *fibrillating*, or quivering, rather than contracting. Again, the AV node plays an important role in filtering some of the electrical activity of the atria—only some of the impulses will be conducted to the ventricles. The resulting ECG tracing will show a baseline that is never smooth or flat, but uneven, reflecting the erratic contractions of the atria. The QRS will look like

**atrial fibrillation:** a heart rhythm that originates from many different locations in the atria and results in atrial activity that is irregular, fast, and chaotic. Some of the irregular atrial impulses are transmitted to the ventricle, which results in fast, irregular QRS complexes and ventricular contractions.

a normal, narrow QRS with a normal duration. The QRS will be conducted at irregular intervals and at a faster rate (100 - 180 bpm) than normal. The QRS will not be preceded by a P wave; no P waves will be present.

Treatment consists of medications and/or electrocardioversion. When atrial fibrillation is treated with medication, the heart rate may return to NSR, or the atrial fibrillation may persist, but with a slower ventricular rate. When atrial fibrillation is present and the heart rate is less than 100 bpm then it is called *atrial fibrillation with controlled ventricular response*. Chronic atrial fibrillation refers to a condition in which atrial fibrillation persists for long periods of time, but the heart rate or ventricular rate is controlled and the patient tolerates the condition well. If the heart rate is over 100 bpm, then it is referred to as *atrial fibrillation with rapid (or uncontrolled) ventricular response*. *New onset atrial fibrillation* is a condition in which atrial fibrillation has started recently and abruptly. When new onset atrial fibrillation occurs, the ventricular response is uncontrolled, with rate ranging from 120 to 180 bpm, and immediate treatment is required.

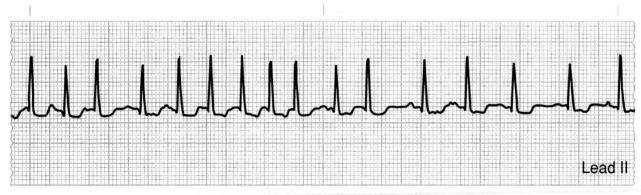

Lead II

**Rate:** 160 bpm. (16 beats in 6 second period; 16 X 10 = bpm.)
**Regularity:** No regular R to R intervals. Irregularly irregular.
**Waveforms:**
   **PR:** No P waves seen. Baseline is irregular and chaotic.
   **QRS:** 0.06 seconds. All QRS complexes look narrow and the same.
Atrial fibrillation with rapid ventricular response.

*Figure 9-4: Atrial Fibrillation with Rapid Ventricular Response*

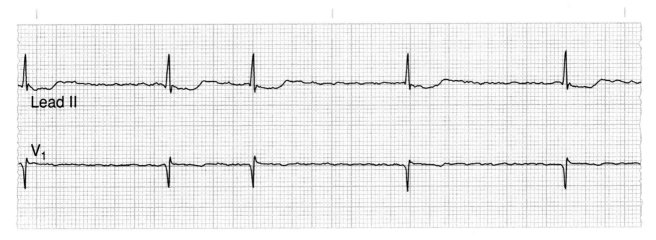

**Rate:** 40- 50 bpm.

**Regularity:** Rhythm is irregular without any pattern.

**Waveforms:**

   **PR:** None. Baseline is irregular with chaotic electrical activity.

   **QRS:** 0.06 seconds. QRS appears irregularly without corresponding P wave.

Atrial activity is disorganized and chaotic. QRS is narrow and occurs irregularly at a slow or controlled rate. This is called a controlled ventricular response because the ventricular rate is not rapid.

*Figure 9-5: Atrial Fibrillation with Controlled Ventricular Response*


## Supraventricular Tachycardia

   **Rate:** 150 – 220 bpm.

   **Regularity:** Usually regular.

   **Waveforms:** The QRS morphology may be the same as NSR or wider.

   • **PR interval:** Usually unable to visualize P waves.

   • **QRS:** 0.04 – 0.14 seconds, may be normal or slightly wider than normal.

*Supraventricular* means above the ventricles. **Supraventricular tachycardia** (SVT) means that the origin of the electrical impulse is above the ventricles, but it cannot be determined if the impulse originates in the atria or in the AV junction. Usually it is not possible to distinguish any P waves so it cannot be called atrial tachycardia. The QRS can be normal, or it can be wider than usual. A wider than normal QRS is referred to as an *aberrantly conducted beat*. This means that the atrial impulse travels down through the AV node as usual. But, instead of traveling down the bundle branches, the impulses travel to the ventricles by an alternate route outside of the bundle branches. In differentiating

**supraventricular tachycardia:** a very rapid, relatively regular heart rhythm that originates above the ventricles, either in the AV junction or atria, and is characterized by difficult to distinguish P waves and a possibly widened QRS.

atrial fibrillation from SVT, remember that atrial fibrillation is very irregular and impulses come from different places in the atria. SVT is more regular, tends to be faster, and usually comes from just one area in the atria or in the AV junction. Many times, a definitive diagnosis cannot be made and a special procedure, called an electrophysiologic test (EPS), is required. If the location of the SVT can be found with the EPS test, then that small area can be burned in a procedure called *radiofrequency ablation,* which prevents the tachycardia from recurring. In this procedure, an electrode is used to deliver a low-voltage, high frequency current to burn and destroy the abnormal tissue that is causing the arrythmia. This eliminates the extra pathway and allows the electrical current to flow down just one pathway, avoiding the condition that allows for a rapid heart rate to develop and persist. SVT can be confused with ventricular tachycardia. The differences between SVT and VT will be discussed later in this chapter.

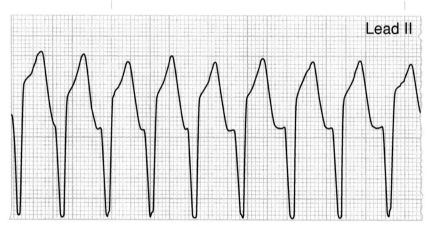

**Rate:** SVT rate, 120 - 140 bpm.

**Regularity:** SVT is regular initially, then slightly irregular.

**Waveforms:**

    **PR:** Not visible.

    **QRS:** 0.12 seconds.

    Rapid rate with a wide QRS (width between 0.11 - 0.14) and rhythm slightly irregular, favors SVT. This means that the rhythm originates above the ventricle, but the exact location is difficult to pinpoint.

*Figure 9-6: Supraventricular Tachycardia (SVT)*

# Junctional Arrhythmias

Arrhythmias that arise from the AV junction are called junctional arrhythmias. The AV node, at the bottom of the right atrium, can slow down impulses or block impulses from traveling to the ventricles. The AV node cannot generate a rhythm, but the surrounding AV junctional tissue can. The AV junction refers to the cardiac tissue where the ventricles and the atria meet. Some junctional arrhythmias are caused by an area of irritable tissue in the AV junction just as some atrial arrhythmias are caused by an area of irritable tissue in the atria. Other junctional arrhythmias occur as a rescue mechanism when the more dominant pacemakers in the heart, such as the SA node, are not working.

## Premature Junctional Contractions (PJC)

**Rate:** 60 – 100 bpm.

**Regularity:** Irregular.

**Waveforms:** The P wave of the premature beat may be retrograde (backward), inverted, or shorter than the normal P wave.

- **PR interval:** The PR of the underlying rhythm is normal.

- **PR interval of the premature beat:** Not present (hidden in the QRS); behind the QRS; inverted (upside down); or if present, < 0.12 seconds.

- **QRS:** 0.04 – 0.10 seconds.

**Premature junctional contraction** is a premature beat generated in the junctional tissue. Because the beat arises in the junctional tissue between the atria and ventricle, the P wave that may arise from this contraction has special characteristics. An electrical impulse originating in the junction will travel from the junction to the atria in a retrograde (backward) manner and at the same time travel antegrade (forward) to the ventricles. Therefore, the atria and the ventricles may depolarize at the same time or at nearly the same time. If they depolarize at the same time, then the P wave will be buried in the QRS. If they depolarize at nearly the same time, then the P wave may be noticed after the QRS. So, the P wave may come after the QRS or, if it precedes the QRS, it will be shorter than normal or inverted (upside down). The QRS will be normal.

**premature junctional contraction (PJC):** an early heart beat that originates in the AV junctional tissue as a result of irritability and travels retrograde (backward) to the atria and antegrade (forward) to the ventricles.

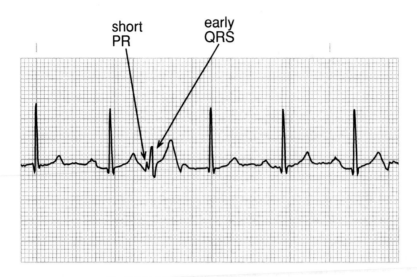

**Rate:** 80 bpm.

**Regularity:** Regular with early (premature) beat (3rd beat).

**Waveforms:**

    **PR:** 0.22 seconds in sinus beat. PR of premature beat is 0.06 seconds.

    **QRS:** 0.06 seconds in sinus beat and premature beat.

The premature beat originates in the AV junction so that it travels retrograde (backward) up to the atria and antegrade (forward) to the ventricles. This means that the atria are depolarized at the same time as, or a little before, the ventricles. The P wave is short because it is partially obscured by the QRS. In the case of PJCs, the P wave can be short, invisibly hidden within the QRS, or after the QRS.

*Figure 9-7: Premature Junctional Contraction (PJC)*

## Junctional Escape

    **Rate:** 40 – 60 bpm.

    **Rhythm:** Regular.

    **Waveforms:** The QRS morphology is similar to that of NSR.

        • **PR interval:** Not present (hidden in the QRS); behind the QRS; inverted; or if present, < 0.12 seconds.

        • **QRS:** 0.04 – 0.10 seconds.

**junctional escape:** a back up pacing rhythm that will take over when other pacemakers, like the SA node, fail.

**Junctional escape** rhythm is a rescue rhythm. If the SA node does not function by discharging an electrical impulse to depolarize the atria and ventricles, then the AV junction has the capability of acting like a back up pacemaker. When a more dominant pacemaker is not functioning, then the AV junction will generate the electrical impulse and keep the heart going. The heart is such an important organ that it has back up processes. Of course, the junctional rate may be too slow, and the patient may feel weak or lightheaded. Because the junctional rate is slow, when the SA node functions properly the AV junction will not compete with it for the pacemaker function. Its purpose is solely as a back up. It is better to have a slow rhythm than no rhythm at all, but the underlying cause for the SA node dysfunction must be found. A drug may be responsible for a dramatic slowing of the SA node that allows the AV junction a chance to emerge as pacemaker. If the SA node is permanently damaged, then an artificial pacemaker may be required to maintain an adequate heart rate.

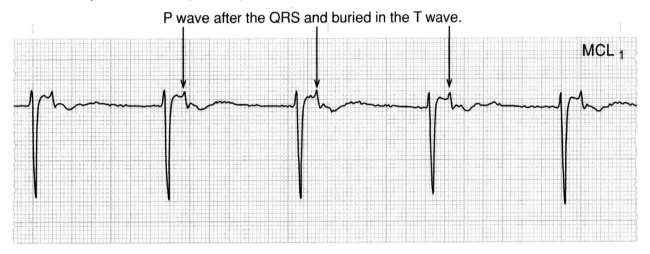

P wave after the QRS and buried in the T wave.

**Rate:** 45 bpm.
**Regularity:** Rhythm is regular.
**Waveforms:**
   **PR:** Cannot measure. P wave is retrograde, or after the QRS.
   **QRS:** 0.10 sec.
The junction fires at the rate of 40 - 60 bpm. So, a junctional escape rhythm usually falls within 40 - 60 bpm. The P wave is either short, hidden in the QRS, or after the QRS. Junctional escape occurs when higher pacemakers, such as the SA node, fail.

*Figure 9-8: Junctional Escape*

Sometimes junctional rhythm can be accelerated, or faster, than the expected 40 - 60 bpm. When this happens, it may look similar to the Figure 9-9.

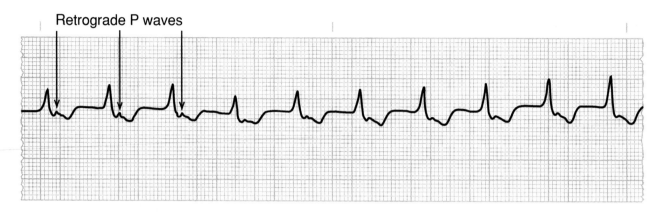

Rate: 100 bpm.

Regularity: Regular.

Waveforms:

PR: Cannot measure. P wave is retrograde to the QRS.

QRS: 0.08 seconds.

P wave is retrograde so this is a junctional rhythm. But, since the heart rate is 100 bpm, faster than expected (Junctional rhythm is usually 40 - 65 bpm.), it is referred to as an *accelerated junctional rhythm*.

*Figure 9-9: Accelerated Junctional Rhythm*

# Ventricular Arrhythmias

Ventricular arrhythmias arise from the ventricular tissue. They range from insignificant disturbances to life-threatening conditions.

### Premature Ventricular Contraction (PVC)

**Rate:** 60 – 100 bpm (underlying rhythm).

**Regularity:** Irregular, with a compensatory pause.

**Waveforms:** PR, P wave, and QRS of underlying rhythm are normal.

- **PR interval of premature beat:** Doesn't exist.

- **QRS of premature beat:** > 0.12, wide, bizarre, and the T wave may be inverted or go in the opposite direction from the QRS of the premature beat.

**premature ventricular contraction (PVC):** an early heart beat that originates in the ventricle as a result of ventricular irritability.

The **premature ventricular contraction**, or (**PVC**), is an early beat that originates in the ventricle. As with other premature beats, PVCs occur because of irritable tissue, in this case irritable tissue in the ventricles. The PVC is generated in the ventricle and then proceeds to spread out as a wave of depolarization that moves from one originating point in the ventricle to the rest of the ventricular tissue. When the electrical impulse travels from the SA node, to the AV node, to the bundle branches, and then to the ventricles, the depolarization is swift and efficient. But, when the impulse travels from a point in the ventricular tissue to the rest of the ventricle, the impulse does not have the benefit of the quick and organized depolarization provided by the bundle branches. As a result, the depolarization occurs slowly, creating a wide QRS with a bizarre form; the QRS complex is wider and may have extra angular markings. The repolarization also becomes abnormal, making the T wave look unusual; the T wave will usually form in the opposite direction of the QRS. This type of wave is called an inverted T wave.

A compensatory pause after the abnormal beat's QRS will confirm that the premature beat is ventricular. The presence of a compensatory pause is easy to determine. Locate the premature beat. Set your calipers to the R to R interval prior to the appearance of the abnormal beat. With the calipers set to this interval, place one arm at the beat just prior to the abnormal beat. The second arm of the caliper will fall beyond the point of the R wave of the abnormal beat and there will be no beat where the arm falls. Pivot the caliper on the second arm and flip the first arm to measure out one more R to R interval. The arm should fall right on the next R wave that occurs after the abnormal beat. In other words, the interval from the last normal beat to the next normal beat after the premature beat should be exactly two R to R cycles. The premature beat creates a refractory period in which the normal beat cannot be conducted at the designated interval (one R to R cycle). The SA node does not reset itself and the next normal beat comes in at the same time as it would if there had not been a PVC. The visual effect is that there is an irregularity involving the premature beat and then a slight pause after the PVC.

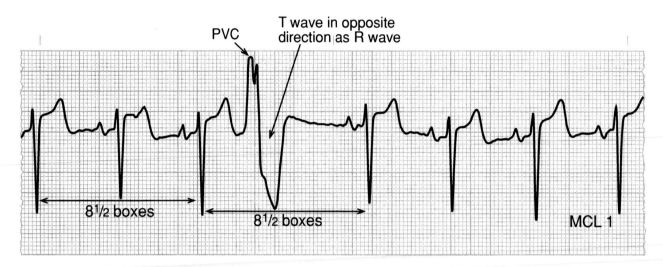

**Rate:** 70 bpm.
**Regularity:** Regular
**Waveforms:**
   **PR:** 0.20 seconds.
   **QRS:** 0.10 seconds in sinus beat. 0.20 seconds in PVC
PVC is wide, 0.20 seconds, in the opposite direction of the sinus beat, and has a T wave in the opposite direction. Also, a compensatory pause is present. This means that two R to R cycles will equal the length of time between the R wave before the PVC and the R wave after the PVC. In this case, two R to R cycles is approximately 8$^{1}$/$_{2}$ large boxes.

*Figure 9-10: Premature Ventricular Contraction (PVC)*

Occasional PVCs may be present without presenting a threat to the patient. However, frequent PVCs may trigger ventricular tachycardia, which is a significant threat to the stability of the patient. Similar to PACs, PVCs can occur in frequent patterns. **Ventricular bigeminy** refers to a pattern consisting of PVCs alternating with sinus beats; every other beat is a PVC. **Ventricular trigeminy** is when PVCs occur every third beat. This will give the appearance of a regularly irregular rhythm pattern. If more than one area of the ventricles is irritable, then there may be PVCs from these different areas. The PVCs from different parts of the ventricle may have different forms. Both PVCs will be wide and bizarre, but the formation and deflection may be different. When two different-looking PVCs are present, they are called **multifocal PVCs**.

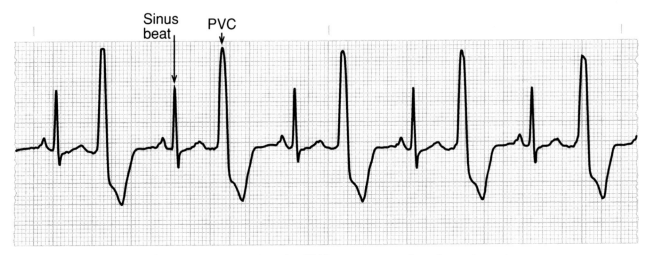

**Rate:** 100 bpm. is the rate if the ECG strip, but the PVCs may not perfuse (meaning not much blood is ejected from the heart when the contraction results from a PVC). So the pulse in the periphery (such as the pulse obtained at the radial artery in the wrist) may be different. The sinus beats may be the only beats that generate a pulse, so the pulse may be only 50 bpm.

**Regularity:** Rhythm is irregular, but in a pattern. This is called *regularly irregular.*

**Waveforms:**

   **PR:** 0.16 seconds There is a P wave for sinus beats (about half the beats).

   **QRS:** 0.08 seconds in the sinus beats. 0.12 seconds in the PVCs.

You can distinguish the sinus beats because they have a P wave and a narrow QRS. The PVCs are wide and do not have a QRS. The PVCs occur every other beat; this is called *ventricular bigeminy.*

*Figure 9-11: Ventricular Bigeminy*

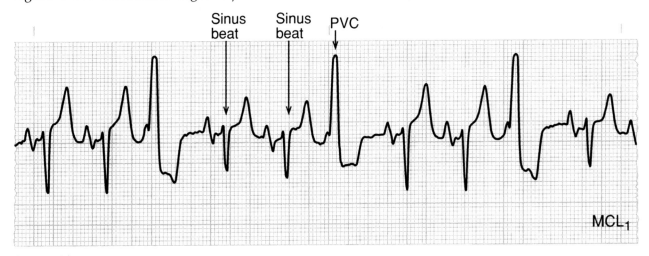

**Rate:** 95 bpm.

**Regularity:** Irregular, but in a pattern. So, regularly irregular.

**Waveforms:**

   **PR:** 0.20 seconds.

   **QRS:** 0.10 seconds in sinus beat. 0.12 seconds in PVC.

The PVCs occur every third beat; is called *ventricular trigeminy.*

*Figure 9-12: Ventricular Trigeminy*

## Ventricular Tachycardia

**Rate:** 100 – 200 bpm.

**Regularity:** Regular.

**Waveform:** The QRS morphology is wider and more bizarre than that of NSR.

- **PR interval:** P waves are not visible, or if they are visible, then they are dissociated from the QRS. There is not a P wave for every QRS.

- **QRS:** > 0.12, wide and bizarre.

**ventricular tachycardia:** a rapid run of PVCs in a row without any sinus beats.

**Ventricular tachycardia** (VT) is a tachycardia that originates in the ventricles. VT is many PVCs in a row without any sinus beats. The manner in which the electrical impulse is transmitted to the ventricles is disorganized and not very effective. The resulting mechanical contraction of the ventricle will not be very effective either. This can produce an unstable blood pressure and can be a life-threatening condition. Sometimes VT can occur in short bursts of 5 to 20 beats. If the tachycardia terminates spontaneously, then no immediate interventions are required. However, if VT is sustained or prolonged, then emergency medications and procedures must be initiated to correct the problem.

As mentioned earlier, it may be difficult to distinguish VT from SVT with a wide QRS. A few guidelines may be helpful to distinguish between the two rhythms:

- If the QRS is less wide, that is, in the range of 0.12 – 0.14 seconds, this favors SVT.

- If the QRS is > 0.14, this favors VT.

- If dissociated P waves can be detected, then a diagnosis of VT is favored. "Dissociated P waves" means that the atria are beating separately from the ventricles and P waves can be identified only sporadically, not at regular intervals. In other words, there would not be a P wave for every QRS in VT. In SVT, P waves are not present (depending on where it originates from) or, if present, are not detectable.

If the patient is stable, a 12-Lead ECG may be needed for further information. Sometimes it takes an expert to correctly tell the difference between SVT and VT.

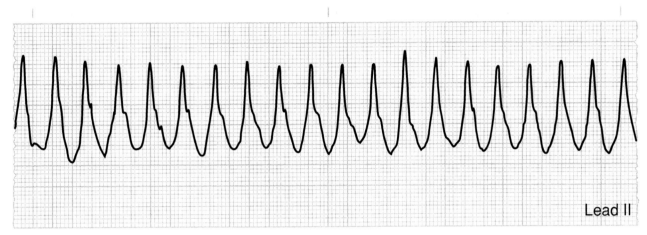

Lead II

**Rate:** 180 bpm.

**Regularity:** Rhythm is regular.

**Waveforms:**

   **PR:** None.

   **QRS:** 0.20 seconds - very wide.

Many PVCs in a row is called ventricular tachycardia. This means that the electrical impulse starts in the ventricles and spreads throughout the heart. The QRS is wide because the electrical impulse is traveling through the ventricles and bypassing the fast track bundle branches. The ventricle does not pump effectively when stimulated in this way, and the fast rate does not allow the ventricles to fill with blood. Therefore, this rhythm does not produce and adequate cardiac output or adequate blood pressure. This creates an unstable condition and constitutes a medical emergency.

*Figure 9-13: Ventricular Tachycardia (VT)*

## Ventricular Fibrillation

   **Rate:** Indeterminate.

   **Regularity:** Chaotic, disorganized.

   **Waveforms:** No waveforms are distinguishable.

   • **PR interval:** None.

   • **QRS:** None; no organized ventricular activity.

Ventricular tachycardia can deteriorate into **ventricular fibrillation** if not treated. Ventricular fibrillation is a life-threatening condition. There is no organized atrial or ventricular activity. The ventricles are quivering and are unable to contract in an organized, coordinated manner. Since the ventricles are not contracting, there is no blood pressure. Immediate intervention is required—either by CPR or by defibrillation. Defibrillation is a procedure in which the patient is given an electrical shock to the chest in order to stimulate the heart to beat normally. The electrical shock attempts to depolarize the heart

**ventricular fibrillation:** a life-threatening condition in which there is no organized atrial or ventricular activity, and the ventricles are quivering and unable to contract.

muscle in an effort to get the heart muscle's own coordinated electrical activity reestablished. Ventricular fibrillation looks like an erratic uneven line on the ECG. There are no recognizable waveforms or complexes. It looks like disorganized electrical activity.

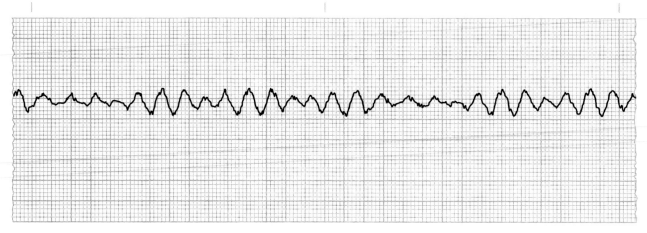

The baseline shows disorganized and chaotic electrical activity. No discernible waveforms are detected. The heart will not be able to produce a blood pressure with this disorganized rhythm.

This is a medical emergency.

*Figure 9-14: Ventricular Fibrillation*

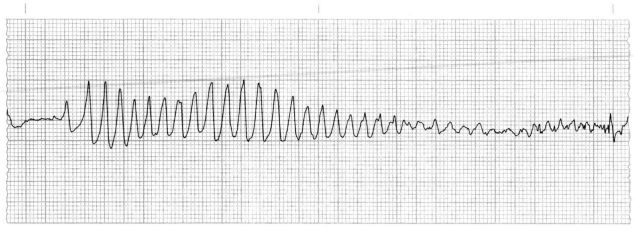

Ventricular tachycardia which quickly deteriorates into ventricular fibrillation in the last half of the strip.

Notice how the electrical activity is disorganized and chaotic. There are no distinct or measurable waveforms.

This is a medical emergency.

*Figure 9-15: Ventricular Rhythms*

## Idioventricular Rhythm

**Rate:**  40 beats per minute.

**Regularity:** Usually regular.

**Waveforms:** The QRS morphology is wider and bizarre when compared to the QRS of NSR.

- **PR interval:** None.

- **QRS:** > 0.12 seconds.

If both the SA node and the AV junction fail, the final back up pacemaker is the ventricle. In the event of an SA node and AV junction failure, the ventricle will pace the heart in a rhythm known as **idioventricular rhythm**, or ventricular escape rhythm. The idioventricular rhythm produces a very slow rate (less than 40 bpm) so that it will not compete with the more dominant pacemakers when they are functioning. As stated previously, it is better to have a slow rhythm than no rhythm at all; this is a rescue rhythm. Since the electrical stimulus is coming from the ventricle, and it is not being transmitted through the bundle branches. This makes the QRS wider than normal. A patient will be unable to tolerate such a slow heart beat for very long, so emergency interventions will be necessary; either medications or an artificial pacemaker will need to be implanted to restore the beat to NSR.

**idioventricular rhythm:**
a back up pacing rhythm that comes from the ventricles when higher pacemakers fail.

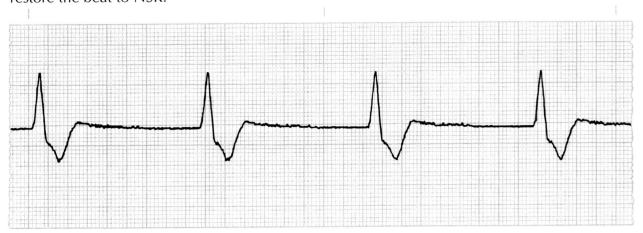

**Rate:** 35 bpm. (8<sup>1/2</sup> large boxes)
**Regularity:** Regular.
**Wavefoms:**
  **PR:** None.
  **QRS:** 0.14 seconds.
Slow, wide QRS indicates that this is a ventricular escape rhythm. Rhythms such as these indicate that higher pacemakers such as the SA node or the AV junction have failed, requiring the ventricle to act as a back-up pacemaker.

*Figure 9-16: Idioventricular Rhythm or Ventricular Escape*

# Heart Block

Heart blocks, or conduction, disturbances are characterized by defects in the conduction system that delay, or block, the electrical impulse traveling through the heart. There are three degrees of atrioventricular heart block: first, second, and third. Second degree AV heart block is further subdivided into Mobitz Type I and Mobitz Type II.

### First Degree AV Heart Block

**first degree AV heart block:** a disturbance in the electrical activity of the heart in which the PR interval is prolonged and the rest of the ECG waveforms are within normal limits.

**Rate:** 60 – 100 bpm.

**Regularity:** Regular.

**Waveforms**: The QRS morphology will be normal.

- **PR interval:** Prolonged, > 0.20 seconds.

- **QRS:** 0.04 – 0.12 seconds.

**First degree AV heart block** is simply characterized by a prolonged PR interval. Every other parameter is within the normal limits.

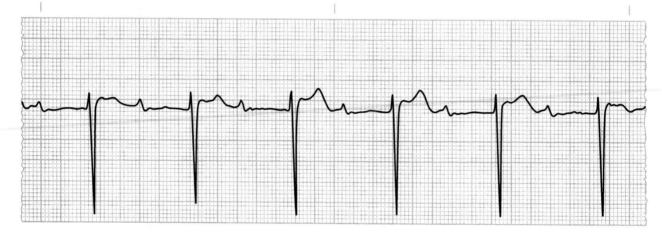

**Rate:** 58 bpm.
**Regularity:** Regular.
**Waveforms:**
    **PR:** 0.56 seconds
    **QRS:** 0.10 seconds
Prolonged PR interval greater than 0.20 seconds indicates first degree AV block.

*Figure 9-17: First Degree AV Heart Block*

## Second Degree AV Heart Block: Mobitz Type I (Wenckebach)

**Rate:** 60 – 100 bpm (probably at the lower end of the range).

**Regularity:** Irregular.

**Waveforms:** There will not be a QRS for every P wave (there will be more P waves than QRSs).

- **PR interval:** Progressively lengthens until a QRS is dropped.

- **QRS:** 0.04 – 0.10 seconds.

**Second degree AV heart block: Mobitz Type I** is also called "**Wenckebach's phenomenon.**" It is characterized by a progressive lengthening of the PR interval until a QRS is dropped. The progressive lengthening may be difficult to determine at first. At first glance the rhythm will look irregular. Remember to track all the P waves to see if there is a QRS for every P wave. Then it will become evident if a QRS is missing. This dropping of a QRS occurs in a cyclical pattern. In other words, there will be a certain number of beats (1 beat = a P wave followed by a QRS), and then a dropped QRS. Then the pattern is repeated. For example, a QRS may be dropped every fourth beat. Identifying this pattern may be tricky at first; just remember to be observant and to analyze the rhythm systematically.

> **second degree AV heart block (Mobitz Type I):** a disturbance in the electrical activity of the heart that involves a gradual lengthening of the PR interval until a QRS is dropped. Also called Wenckebach.

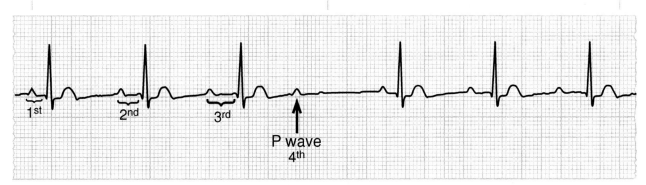

**Rate:** 60 bpm.
**Regularity:** Irregular.
**Waveforms:**
  **PR:** Progressive lengthening until QRS is dropped.
        1st PR: 0.18 seconds
        2nd PR: 0.22 seconds
        3rd PR: 0.30 seconds
        4th PR: QRS is dropped
  **QRS:** 0.08 seconds
There is not a QRS for every P wave. More P waves exist than QRSs. The progressive lengthening of the PR interval is the hallmark of Wenckebach.

*Figure 9-18: Second Degree AV Heart Block: Mobitz Type 1 (Wenckebach)*

## Second Degree AV Heart Block: Mobitz Type II

**second degree AV heart block (Mobitz Type II):** a disturbance in the electrical activity of the heart in which an intermittent block between the atrial and ventricular conduction systems results in randomly dropped QRSs and more P waves than QRSs. A high degree of block would result in more blocked QRSs and a slower heart rate.

**Rate:** 40 – 100 bpm.

**Regularity:** Irregular.

**Waveforms:** The P waves will march out regularly, but QRSs will be irregular; randomly there will be a dropped QRS. There will be more P waves than QRSs.

- **PR interval:** Can be prolonged or within normal limits.
- **QRS:** 0.04 – 0.10 seconds.

With **second degree AV heart block: Mobitz Type II** the SA node will generate an impulse, but the impulse will randomly not be conducted to the ventricle, resulting in a dropped QRS. This will be evident by the regular appearance of P waves followed by QRSs, except that at random points within the normal pattern a P wave will appear without a corresponding QRS. There is no pattern or regularity as to when a QRS will be dropped. Initially the patient will be stable, but as the conduction defect worsens there will be more dropped (blocked) QRSs. Eventually the patient may need a pacemaker to correct the defect.

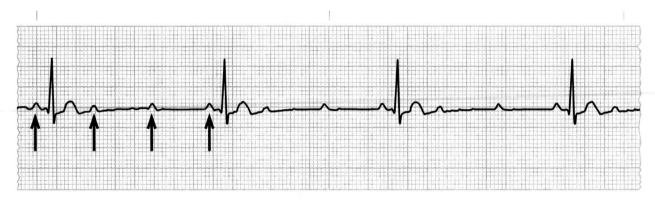

**Rate:** Atrial – P waves occur at a rate of 100 bpm.
　　　　Ventricular – QRS occurs at a rate of 35 bpm.
**Regularity:** Atrial and ventricular rhythms are regular.
**Waveforms:**
　　**PR:** 0.16 seconds
　　**QRS:** 0.08 seconds
More P waves are present than QRSs. The PR interval is constant at 0.16 seconds when conducted to the ventricle. The electrical impulse is suddenly blocked and the QRS dropped. There are three P waves for every QRS. This is called 3:1 Block.

*Figure 9-19: Second Degree AV Heart Block: Mobitz Type II*

## Third Degree AV Heart Block

**Rate:** < 60 bpm.

**Regularity:** May be regular or irregular.

**Waveforms:** The atria and the ventricles are beating separately and independently. The P wave and the QRS occur regularly, but at different rates.

- **PR interval:** The P wave may be obscured by the QRS, making the PR interval difficult to locate.

- **QRS:** May be wide or normal width.

**Third degree AV heart block** means that there is a complete heart block between the atria and the ventricles. Impulses originating in the SA node are unable to travel to the ventricles. The result is that the atria beat independently from the ventricles. A P wave may be detected throughout the rhythm strip, appearing at regular intervals and at a normal rate. There will not be a P wave for every QRS; and no P wave will be conducted to the ventricle to produce a QRS. The QRS will be regular, but it will appear at a slower rate than the P wave, and out of synchronicity with the P wave because it is being generated by the ventricles.

**third degree AV heart block:** a complete block between the atria and the ventricles so that the atria beat independently from the ventricles.

Because the impulses from the SA node are unable to travel to the ventricles, a junctional escape or an idioventricular rhythm will take over the pacemaker duties for the ventricle. The type of back-up rhythm that is initiated depends on where the conduction block occurs. If the conduction block occurs at the AV node, then the AV junction will establish a junctional escape rhythm. Remember that the junctional escape will have a narrow QRS and a heart rate of 40 – 60 bpm. If the conduction block occurs below the AV node, then an idioventricular rhythm will take over. The idioventricular rhythm will have a wide QRS and a rate of less than 40 bpm. So the SA node may produce a P wave at a rate of 75 bpm, without conduction to the ventricles; and the ventricles may beat at a rate of 30 – 40 bpm completely independent from the atrial contraction. Usually, an artificial pacemaker is inserted to treat third degree AV heart block.

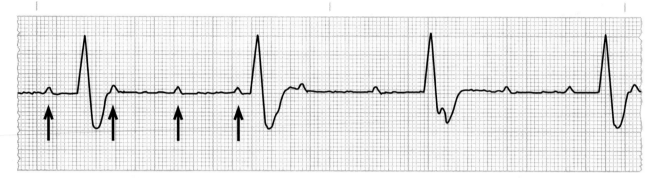

**Rate:** Atrial - 95 bpm.
        Ventricular - 35 bpm.
**Regularity:** Atrial and ventricular rhythms are regular.
**Waveforms:**
 **PR:** None.
 **QRS:** 0.16 sec.
P waves occur at a regular interval and are dissociated with the occurrence of the QRSs. The atria (P waves) and the ventricles (QRSs) are beating independently. None of the P waves are conducted to the ventricles to cause a QRS. This is complete heart block, or third degree HB. Since the QRS is wide, it is a ventricular escape rhythm.

*Figure 9-20: Third degree AV Heart Block with Ventricular Escape Rhythm*

## Bundle Branch Block

**Rate:** 60 – 100 bpm.

**Regularity:** Regular.

**Waveforms:** There is a P wave for every QRS.

- **PR interval:** 0.12 – 0.20 seconds.

- **QRS:** 0.12 seconds.

**bundle branch block (BBB):** a block in one of the bundle branches that prolongs the time it takes for the electrical impulse to travel from the ventricular septum to the rest of the ventricles, resulting in a widened QRS.

The QRS is wide when a **bundle branch block** (BBB) is present. The block may be in the right or the left bundle branch. In most cases, the bundle branch that contains the blockage will not be able to be determined from the rhythm strip. Usually, a 12-Lead ECG will be needed in order to determine if the blockage is in the right or left bundle branch. Rhythm strips reflecting an $MCL_1$ or $V_1$ lead are used to distinguish between right and left bundle branch blocks. In $MCL_1$ or $V_1$, if the QRS is wide and positive, then it is a right bundle branch block; if the QRS is wide and negative, then it is a left bundle branch block.

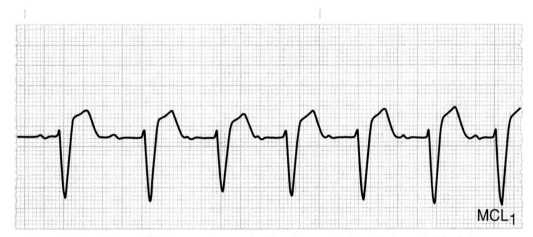

In $V_1$ or $MCL_1$, if the QRS is negative and wide, then a left bundle branch block is present. In this example, the QRS measures 0.16 seconds.

*Figure 9-21: Left Bundle Branch Block*

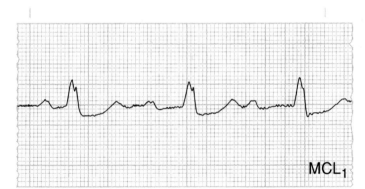

In lead $V_1$ or $MCL_1$, if the QRS is wide and upright, then a right bundle branch block is present. The QRS in this example is 0.12 seconds.

*Figure 9-22: Right Bundle Branch Block*

# Other Significant Rhythms

## Pacemaker Rhythm

**Rate:** Variable, usually 60 – 100 bpm.

**Regularity:** Regular.

**Waveforms:** The QRS will be wide and squared-off.

- **PR interval:** Normal, or may have a pacer spike.

- **QRS:** Will be wider than normal and is preceded by a pacer spike.

**pacemaker rhythm:**
an ECG tracing characterized by definite spikes before the P wave and/ or QRS which represent the action of an artificial pace- maker.

Pacemakers are placed into patients who are experiencing either heart block or a heart rate that is too slow. These devices generate a **pacemaker rhythm**. Pacemakers usually work within a specified range. The lower limit is usually set at 60 bpm so that the patient's heart rate will never go below 60. Many pacemakers are rate responsive. So, if a patient is performing an activity and needs a higher heart rate, the pacemaker will increase to an upper limit. Usually, this upper limit is not higher than 120 bpm. The ventricles can be paced, and sometimes both the atrium and the ventricles can be paced. It depends on the type of pacemaker that is used and the rate at which the pacemaker is set. The sharp spike at the beginning of a wave indicates that it is a paced beat. If the QRS is paced, it will be wider than normal because the impulse is traveling through the ventricle — not through the bundle branches.

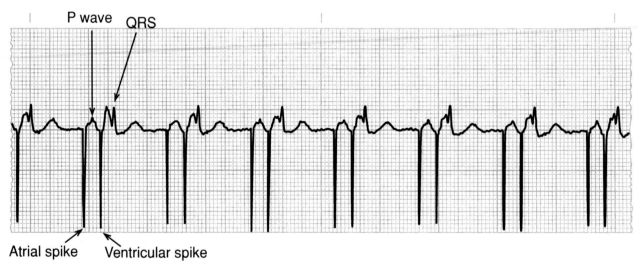

In AV pacing, the atrium and the ventricles are paced in order to mimic the natural function of the heart. The atrial spikes will produce a P wave and the ventricular spike will produce a QRS.

*Figure 9-23: AV (Atrioventricular) Pacing*

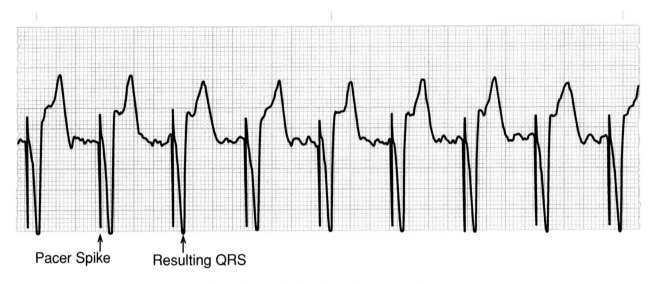

Pacer Spike        Resulting QRS

A pacemaker delivers an electrical impulse to the heart and takes over the pacemaker function when the heart's own pacemaking function fails. On the ECG, the pacemaker activity is recorded as a sharp spike followed by a waveform. In this case, the ventricle is paced so the pacer spike is followed by a QRS.

*Figure 9-24: Ventricular Pacing*

## Aystole

**Rate:** 0 bpm.

**Rhythm:** Straight line.

**Waveform:** No waveforms present, no electrical activity.

**asystole:**
a state in which there is no electrical or mechanical activity occurring in the heart; a "flat line" on the ECG.

Aystole is also called "flat line" or "straightline." No waveforms are present and there is no electrical activity. This is a medical emergency. Medication and CPR must be administered immediately.

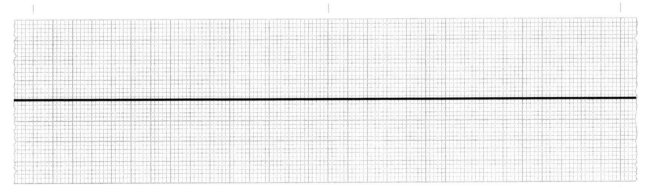

*Figure 9-25: Asystole, No Electrical Activity*

# Chapter Summary

Abnormal rhythms are those that occur outside of the sinus mechanism. Atrial arrhythmias originate in the atria; junctional arrhythmias originate in the AV junction; and ventricular arrhythmias originate in the ventricles. Arrhythmias can occur infrequently and be harmless. But, if arrhythmias are continuous or sustained, the patient will experience symptoms of shortness of breath or light-headedness, and treatment will be required. Some heart rhythms such as ventricular tachycardia, ventricular fibrillation, and asystole are life-threatening conditions that require immediate treatment.

Name_____

Date_____

# Student Enrichment Activities

## <u>Atrial Arrhythmias</u>

**Examine and interpret the rhythm strips below.**

1. • Rate _____     • QRS _____
   • Regularity _____     • Abnormal beats _____
   • PR interval _____     • Interpretation _____

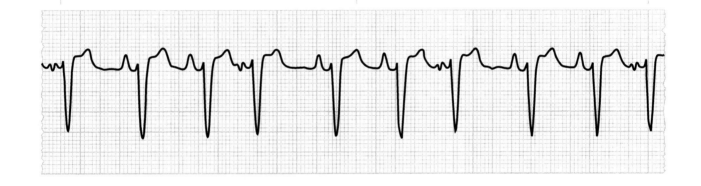

2. • Rate _____     • QRS _____
   • Regularity _____     • Abnormal beats _____
   • PR interval _____     • Interpretation _____

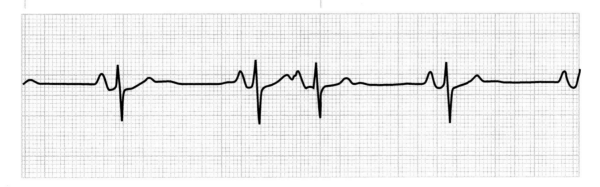

**3.** • Rate _____    • QRS _____

   • Regularity _____    • Abnormal beats _____

   • PR interval _____    • Interpretation _____

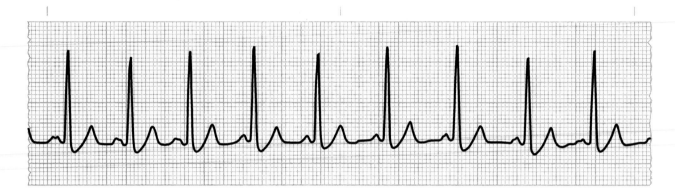

**4.** • Rate _____    • QRS _____

   • Regularity _____    • Abnormal beats _____

   • PR interval _____    • Interpretation _____

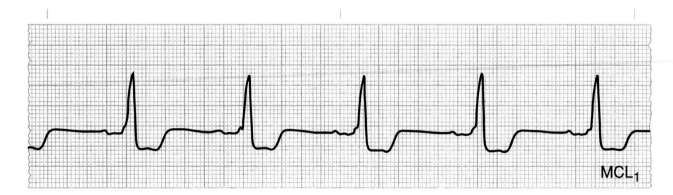

Name_____

Date_____

**5.** • Rate _____          • QRS _____

   • Regularity _____          • Abnormal beats _____

   • PR interval _____          • Interpretation _____

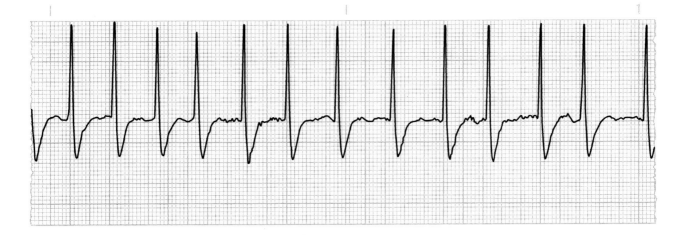

**6.** • Rate _____          • QRS _____

   • Regularity _____          • Abnormal beats _____

   • PR interval _____          • Interpretation _____

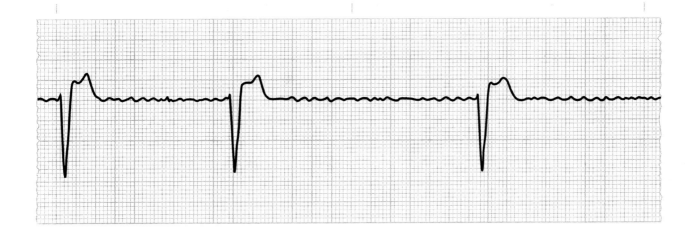

7. • Rate _____     • QRS _____
   • Regularity _____        • Abnormal beats _____
   • PR interval _____       • Interpretation _____

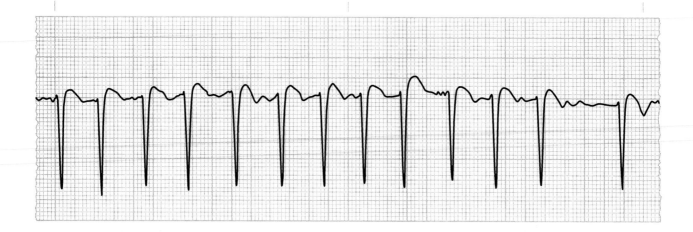

8. • Rate _____     • QRS _____
   • Regularity _____        • Abnormal beats _____
   • PR interval _____       • Interpretation _____

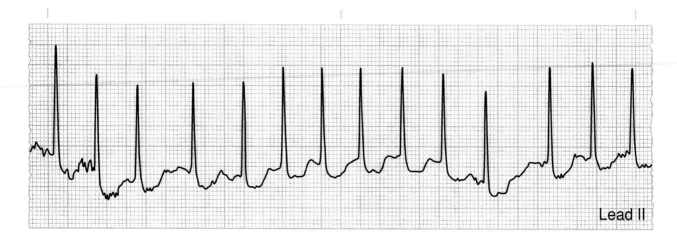

Lead II

Name_____

Date_____

9. • Rate _____    • QRS _____

    • Regularity _____    • Abnormal beats _____

    • PR interval _____    • Interpretation _____

MCL₁

10. • Rate _____    • QRS _____

    • Regularity _____    • Abnormal beats _____

    • PR interval _____    • Interpretation _____

**Complete the following statements.**

11. _____ waves are sawtooth-shaped and occur regularly at a rate of about 300 bpm.

12. In _____ _____ the waveforms are irregular and chaotic.

13. _____ are early beats that interrupt the regular rhythm and are initiated in the atria.

14. PAT stands for _____ _____ _____ and is called this because it _____ and _____suddenly.

15. The atria quiver erratically and have disorganized and chaotic activity during _____ _____.

16. If the ventricular rate of atrial fibrillation is more than 100 bpm, then it is called atrial fibrillation with _____ _____ _____.

17. In atrial flutter, the flutter waves are regular, but the QRS can be irregular because of _____ _____ through the AV node.

18. The AV node protects the ventricle from being bombarded by electrical impulses by _____ some of the impulses during atrial flutter and atrial fibrillation.

19. SVT stands for _____ _____.

20. Supraventricular means _____ the _____.

Name_____

Date_____


21.  SVT can have a wider than normal _____.


22.  SVT can be confused with _____  _____.


23.  _____ _____ is when a PAC occurs every other beat.


24.  When one ventricular beat is conducted for every three flutter waves this is referred to as atrial flutter with _____ _____.


25.  If PACs are present in a heart rhythm, the underlying rhythm is _____.


26.  In atrial fibrillation there are no _____ waves.


## Junctional Arrhythmias

**Examine and interpret the rhythm strips below.**


27.  • Rate _____          • QRS _____

    • Regularity _____          • Abnormal beats _____

    • PR interval _____          • Interpretation _____

**28.**
- Rate _____
- Regularity _____
- PR interval _____

- QRS _____
- Abnormal beats _____
- Interpretation _____

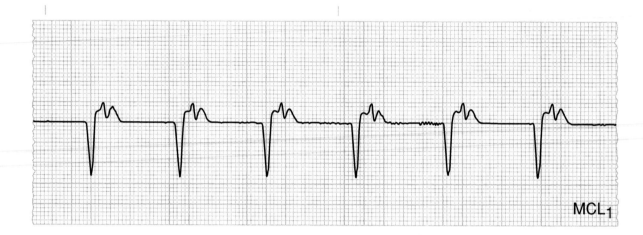

MCL₁

**29.**
- Rate _____
- Regularity _____
- PR interval _____

- QRS _____
- Abnormal beats _____
- Interpretation _____

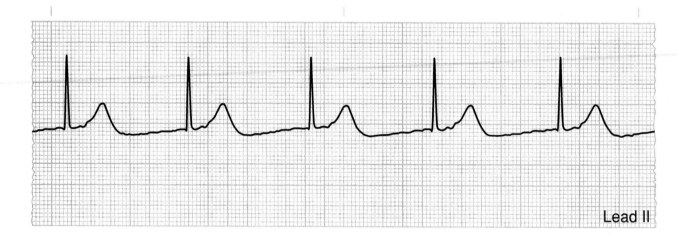

Lead II

Name_____

Date_____

## Complete the following statements.

30. The P wave of a junctional beat can be _____, _____ in the QRS, or _____ the QRS.

31. The P wave of a junctional beat has its unique configuration because it is traveling from the _____ _____ in a _____ manner to the atria.

32. _____ _____ rhythm occurs when the SA node fails to pace the heart.

33. The AV junction protects the heart by acting as a back-up pacemaker and will pace the heart at a rate of _____ to _____ bpm when required.

34. The rate of the AV junction is slow so that it won't compete with the _____ _____ in the pacemaker function.

35. In a junctional beat, the QRS will be _____.

36. When a patient has a junctional rhythm, her or she may experience symptoms such as _____ and/or _____.

## <u>Ventricular Arrhythmias</u>

**Analyze and interpret the below rhythms.**

**37.** • Rate _____   • QRS _____

   • Regularity _____   • Abnormal beats _____

   • PR interval _____   • Interpretation _____

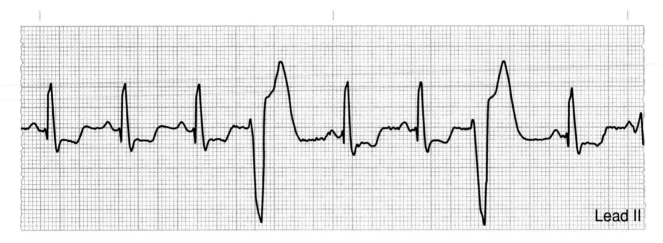

Lead II

**38.** • Rate _____   • QRS _____

   • Regularity _____   • Abnormal beats _____

   • PR interval _____   • Interpretation _____

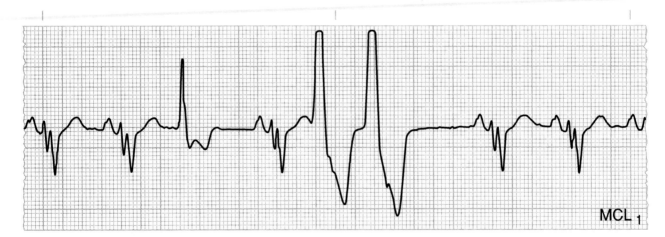

MCL$_1$

Name_____

Date_____

**39.** • Rate _____    • QRS _____

  • Regularity _____    • Abnormal beats _____

  • PR interval _____    • Interpretation _____

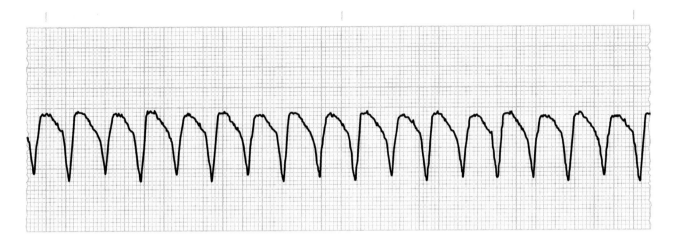

**40.** • Rate _____    • QRS _____

  • Regularity _____    • Abnormal beats _____

  • PR interval _____    • Interpretation _____

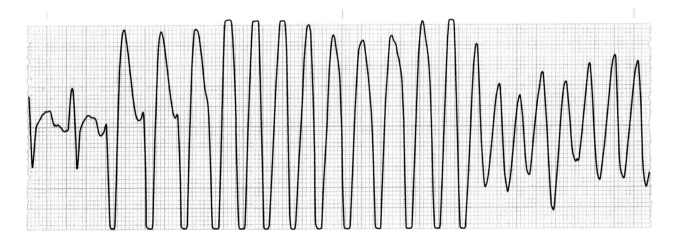

**41.** • Rate _____     • QRS _____

  • Regularity _____     • Abnormal beats _____

  • PR interval _____     • Interpretation _____

Lead II

**42.** • Rate _____     • QRS _____

  • Regularity _____     • Abnormal beats _____

  • PR interval _____     • Interpretation _____

Name_____

Date_____

**43.**  • Rate _____          • QRS _____

    • Regularity _____          • Abnormal beats _____

    • PR interval _____          • Interpretation _____

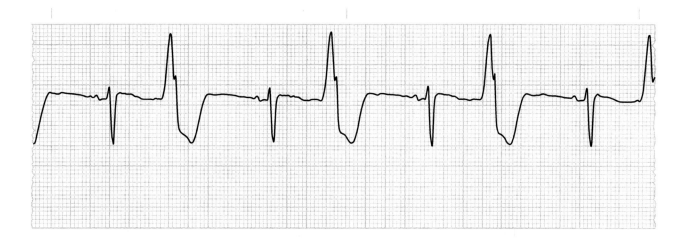

**44.**  • Rate _____          • QRS _____

    • Regularity _____          • Abnormal beats _____

    • PR interval _____          • Interpretation _____

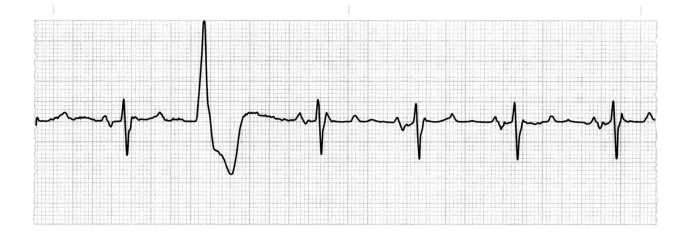

**Complete the following statements.**

45. The QRS of the PVC is early and measures greater than _____.

46. PVCs occurring in a pattern of every other beat are called _____
    _____.

47. PVCs occurring in a pattern of every third beat are called _____
    _____.

48. A _____ _____ is a distinguishing feature of PVCs and refers
    to the pause between the PVC and the next sinus beat.

49. Sustained ventricular tachycardia can last a prolonged period of time. If it isn't
    interrupted, it can be _____.

50. A patient experiencing VT is considered unstable because the heart cannot
    _____ effectively. This requires _____ medications and proce-
    dures to be administered.

51. A diagnosis of VT is favored over a diagnosis of SVT if dissociated _____
    _____ can be detected and the width of the QRS is greater than
    _____.

52. In _____ _____ the heart does not effectively contract, but the
    whole muscle quivers in a disorganized and chaotic manner.

53. A patient in ventricular fibrillation will have no _____ _____.

Name_____

Date_____

## Heart Blocks

**Rhythm analysis and interpretation.**

**54.**
- Rate _____
- Regularity _____
- PR interval _____

- QRS _____
- Abnormal beats _____
- Interpretation _____

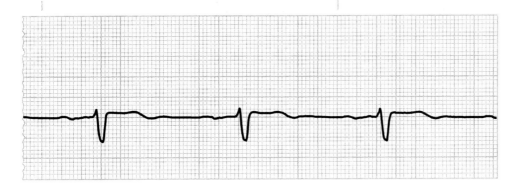

**55.**
- Rate _____
- Regularity _____
- PR interval _____

- QRS _____
- Abnormal beats _____
- Interpretation _____

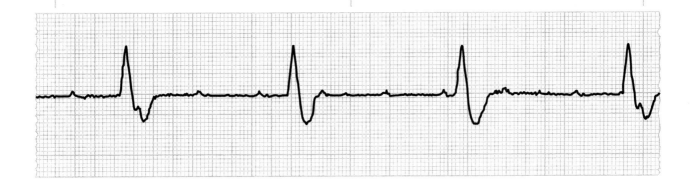

**56.** • Rate _____  • QRS _____

      • Regularity _____  • Abnormal beats _____

      • PR interval _____  • Interpretation _____

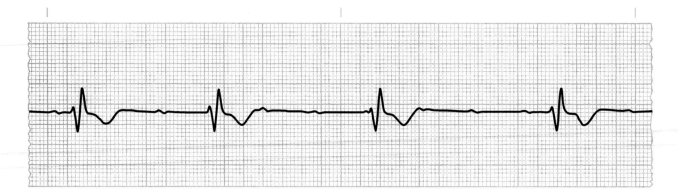

**57.** • Rate _____  • QRS _____

      • Regularity _____  • Abnormal beats _____

      • PR interval _____  • Interpretation _____

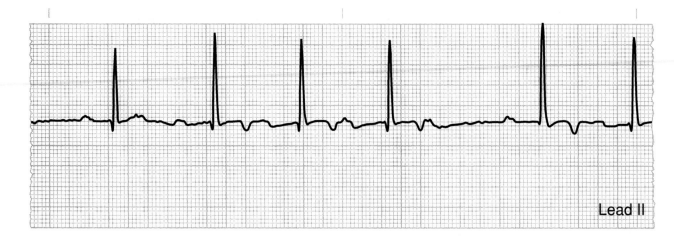

Lead II

Name_____

Date_____

**58.**
- Rate _____
- Regularity _____
- PR interval _____

- QRS _____
- Abnormal beats _____
- Interpretation _____

Lead II

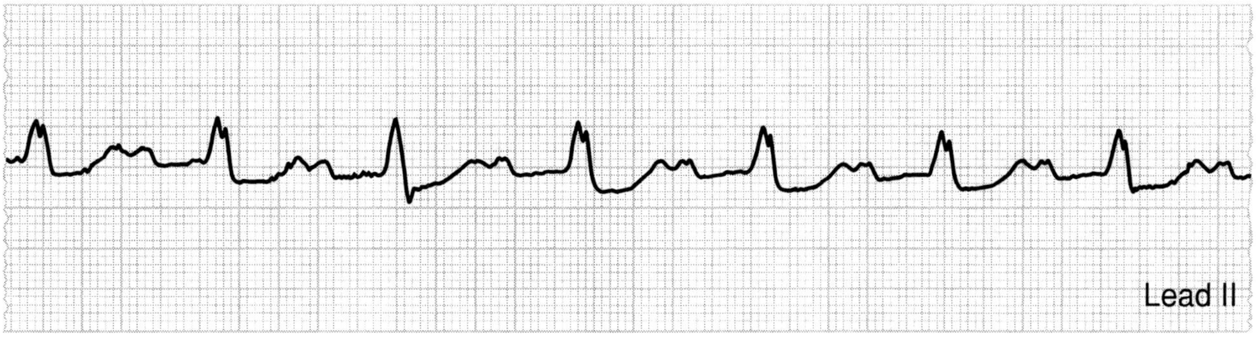

**59.**
- Rate _____
- Regularity _____
- PR interval _____

- QRS _____
- Abnormal beats _____
- Interpretation _____

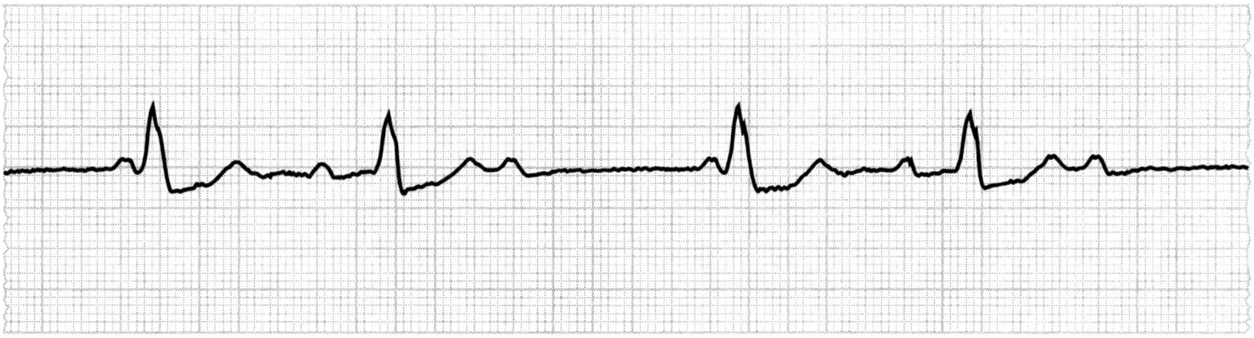

60.  • Rate _____   • QRS _____

   • Regularity _____   • Abnormal beats _____

   • PR interval _____   • Interpretation _____

**Complete the following statements.**

61.  _____ _____ _____ heart block, otherwise called

   _____, is characterized by progressive lengthening of the

   PR interval until a QRS is dropped.

62.  _____ _____ _____ heart block is present when the PR

   interval is longer than normal.

63.  Second degree heart block – Mobitz Type II can be detected by observing a random

   dropping of the _____.

64.  The PR interval in first degree AV heart block measures greater than _____

   seconds.

65.  In second degree AV heart block – Mobitz Type II there are more _____ waves

   than _____.

66.  In second degree AV heart block – Mobitz Type I there are more _____ waves

   than _____.

Name_____

Date_____

**67.** Second degree heart block is _____. (Choose one: regular or irregular.)

**68.** First degree heart block is _____. (Choose one: regular or irregular.)

**69.** In third degree AV heart block the _____ beat independently from the

_____.

**70.** Third degree heart block can have a ventricular contraction caused by

_____ _____ or _____ rhythm.

**71.** Two different types of bundle branch block are_____ and _____.

**72.** The QRS in BBB measures  _____ seconds.

**73.** The overall rhythm of BBB is _____ (Choose one: regular or irregular).

## Other Significant Rhythms

**Analyze the following rhythms.**

**74.**
- Rate _____
- Regularity _____
- PR interval _____
- QRS _____
- Abnormal beats _____
- Interpretation _____

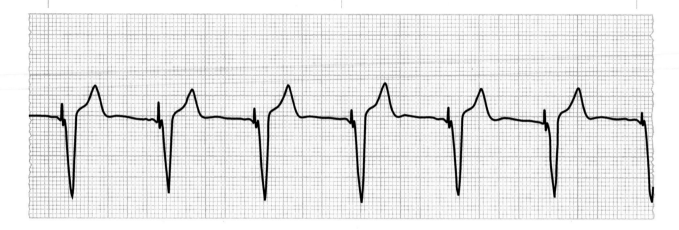

**75.**
- Rate _____
- Regularity _____
- PR interval _____
- QRS _____
- Abnormal beats _____
- Interpretation _____

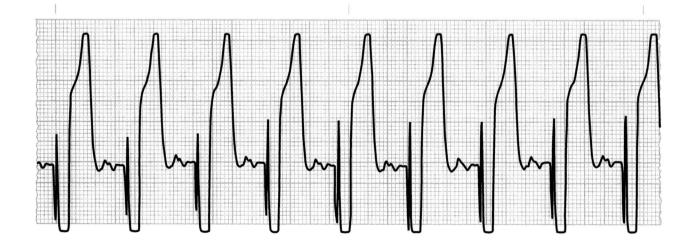

Name_____

Date_____

**Complete the following statements.**

76.  Spikes at the beginning of the waveform are characteristic of a _____

   _____.

77.  A pacemaker can pace the _____ and sometimes both the _____

   and the _____ can be paced.

78.  A pacemaker is necessary if a patient has _____ _____ or a

   heart rate that is too _____.

79.  The rate of the pacemaker is set at a _____ limit and an _____ limit.

80.  The absence of electrical activity is called _____.

# GLOSSARY

**12-Lead ECG:** a tracing of the electrical activity of the heart as viewed from twelve different aspects.

# A

**\*action potential:** the difference in the electrical charge between the two sides of a cell membrane that indicates the probability an electrical current will be discharged.

**acute:** sudden onset; short duration.

**alveoli:** microscopic air sacs within the lungs responsible for the exchange of oxygen and carbon dioxide.

**anatomy:** the study of the structure of the body.

**\*angina:** chest pain caused by decreased blood flow to the heart.

**\*angiogram:** x-rays of arteries after the injection of dye which allows the visualization of the arteries and determination of blockages within the arteries.

**anterior wall:** the front part of the left ventricle that comprises the main portion of the left side of the heart.

**anteroseptal wall:** the area of the heart that extends from the anterior wall to the septum.

**\*aorta:** the large artery that receives blood from the left side of the heart and distributes the blood to the rest of the body.

**\*aortic valve:** the valve on the left side of the heart that opens to allow blood to flow from the left ventricle into the aorta.

**apex:** the bottom, pointed portion of the heart.

**\*arrhythmia:** dysrhythmia; an abnormal heart rhythm.

**\*arteriosclerosis:** thickening and hardening of the arterial walls.

**\*artery:** a blood vessel that carries highly oxygenated blood away from the heart to the tissues.

**\*artifact:** additional electrical activity on an ECG tracing as a result of muscle movement, alternating current (AC), or disruption of the cable, rather than the electrical activity of the heart.

**aspirin:** an over-the-counter drug commonly used to reduce pain, inflammation and fever; widely used to thin the blood and prevent blood clots both during and after a heart attack.

**\*asystole:** a state in which there is no electrical or mechanical activity occurring in the heart; a "flat line" on the ECG.

**atherosclerosis:** narrowing of the arteries caused by fatty build-up within the artery wall and accompanied by a reduction in the artery's ability to dilate and constrict.

**atrial bigeminy:** a heart rhythm in which premature atrial contractions occur every other beat.

**\*atrial fibrillation:** a heart rhythm that originates from many different locations in the atria and results in atrial activity that is irregular, fast, and chaotic. Some of the irregular atrial impulses are transmitted to the ventricle, which results in fast, irregular QRS complexes and ventricular contractions.

**\*atrial flutter:** a heart rhythm that originates from the same location in the atria, resulting in atrial activity that creates a characteristic sawtooth waveform that is very fast. Some of the atrial impulses are transmitted to the ventricles resulting in a fast QRS and ventricular contraction. The QRS may be regular or irregular.

**atrial trigeminy:** a heart rhythm in which premature atrial contractions occur every third beat.

**\*atrioventricular node:** (AV node) special conductive tissue located in the lower right atrium that conducts electrical impulses from the atria to the ventricles.

**\*atrium:** one of the two top chambers of the heart, that receives blood from the large veins and then pumps blood into the lower chambers of the heart.

**augmented voltage:** an increase in voltage with a resulting increase in amplitude that enhances the resulting waveform.

**automaticity:** the unique ability of cardiac muscle to contract spontaneously without outside electrical stimulation.

**AV junction:** The area where the atrium and the ventricle meet.

**axilla:** the armpit.

# B

**\*baseline:** the polarized state in which no perceptible electrical discharge is visible on the ECG; also called the isoelectric line.

**bipolar lead:** a type of lead for which both a positive and a negative sensor are used to view the difference of the electrical energy between these two points and then translate it into a waveform.

**blocked:** obstructed; unable to pass.

**\*blood pressure:** the pressure of the blood exerted against the arteries.

**\*bradycardia:** a pulse rate below 60 beats per minute.

**\*bundle branch block (BBB):** a block in one of the bundle branches that prolongs the time it takes for the electrical impulse to travel from the ventricular septum to the rest of the ventricles, resulting in a widened QRS.

**\*bundle branches:** special conductive tissue fibers that extend from the Bundle of His and into the left and right ventricle.

**\*bundle of His:** special conductive tissue in the middle of the septum of the heart, or interventricular septum, that allows smooth and rapid conduction of the electrical impulse from the AV node to the ventricle.

# C

*cable: one or more insulated wires that connect sensors to an electrocardiograph.
*calibration: the process of setting a machine to a standardized scale so the results will be comparable and tests can be compared.
*calipers: a metal tool used to assist in the accurate measurement of waveforms.
*cardiac: pertaining to the heart.
cardiac cycle: the series of electrical and mechanical events that comprise each heart beat.
*cardiology: the medical specialty which is the study of the heart and diseases of the heart.
*cardiovascular: of or relating to the heart and blood vessels.
*cellular membrane: a layer of protein that surrounds a cell and keeps it separate from the surrounding fluid and cells.
chronic: slow to develop; persisting for a long time.
clavicle: the collar bone.
*conflict resolution: solving problems created by opposing ideas or interests through the use of effective communication and compromise.
congestive heart failure: the inability of the heart to maintain adequate blood circulation.
*coronary arteries: blood vessels that bring oxygen rich blood to the heart muscle.

# D

*depolarization: the period of time when ions or electrolytes are exchanged through a semipermeable membrane and an electrical current is discharged.
diabetic: pertaining to diabetes; a person with diabetes (a disorder of carbohydrate metabolism).
diaphoretic: perspiring excessively.
diaphragm: the dome-shaped muscle separating the thoracic cavity from the abdominal cavity; the portion of the stethoscope used for picking up sound.
*diastole: the period of time when the heart muscle is relaxed.

# E

*electrocardiogram: ECG or EKG; a recording of the electrical activity of the heart. A recording made by an electrocardiograph.
*electrocardiograph: a machine used to record the electrical activity of the heart.
*electrolyte: an ion or a small particle that is positively or negatively charged, such as sodium (Na+), potassium (K+), or chloride (Cl-).
*extracellular: fluid and particles outside of and surrounding the cell.

# F

**filter:** a part of the electrocardiograph used to filter out electrical activity from the environment that may interfere with the electrocardiogram.

**\*first degree AV heart block:** a disturbance in the electrical activity of the heart in which the PR interval is prolonged and the rest of the ECG waveforms are within normal limits.

# G

**gain:** the output of the amplifier.

**\*galvanometer:** a device in the ECG machine which detects electrical currents from a patient and converts it into mechanical energy, which is then recorded onto graph paper.

**glucose:** a simple sugar; used in the human body to produce energy.

**\*graph paper:** paper on which the ECG is recorded that is preprinted with horizontal lines representing time and vertical lines representing voltage.

**\*ground lead:** a lead that is not used to determine electrical activity, but rather as a reference point.

# H

**\*heart block:** a disturbance in the conduction system of the heart.

**\*heart catheterization:** the passage of tubes into the heart for the purpose of diagnosing cardiac disease.

**heart healthy diet:** a term used to describe a low-fat diet containing large amounts of fresh fruits and vegetables, fish or fish oils, and whole grains, and eliminating or minimizing the consumption of red meat.

**\*Holter monitor:** a portable ECG recording machine that a patient wears which records the electrical activity of the heart continuously for 24 to 48 hours.

**horizontal:** moving in the direction of left and/or right, or side to side.

# I

**\*idioventricular rhythm:** a back up pacing rhythm that comes from the ventricles when higher pacemakers fail.

**\*inferior vena cava:** the main vein that drains blood from the lower part of the body into the right atrium of the heart.

**inferior wall:** the bottom portion of the heart that lies over the diaphragm.

**intercostal space:** the area between two successive ribs.

**interval:** the length of a wave with a segment.

**\*intracellular:** within a cell.

**invasive:** describes a procedure in which an instrument or device is inserted into the body.

**irregular:** not regular. Beats that do not occur evenly.

**irregularly irregular:** random irregularity without a pattern.

***ischemia:** decreased blood flow to organs and tissues, such as the heart muscle, caused by the narrowing of the arteries.

***isoelectric line:** the baseline; a straight line on the ECG recording that represents an absence of electrical activity.

# J

***junctional escape:** a back up pacing rhythm that will take over when other pacemakers, like the SA node, fail.

# L

**lateral wall:** the side of the heart that faces the left arm, or left axilla.

***lead:** a configuration of positive and negative sensors, or electrodes, on the body surface that picks up the electrical information from the heart. The different sensor configurations offer different "views" of the heart.

**Lead I:** a view which detects the flow of electrical current through the heart on a plane between the right and left arm that reflects information on the lateral wall of the heart.

**Lead II:** a view which detects the flow of electrical current through the heart on a plane between the right arm and the left leg and that looks up at the heart from the viewpoint of the left leg and reflects information about the inferior wall of the heart.

**Lead III:** a view which detects the flow of electrical current through the heart on a plane between the left arm and left leg and that also looks up at the heart from the viewpoint of the left leg and gives information about the inferior wall of the heart.

**lead selector:** the control on the electrocardiograph that designates which view of the heart will be recorded.

**left atrium:** the upper chamber on the left side of the heart that receives oxygenated blood from the lungs via the pulmonary veins.

**left ventricle:** the lower chamber on the left side of the heart that pumps blood through the aorta into the arteries.

**lipids:** fatty type substances characterized by their insolubility in water that, in high levels, are associated with coronary artery disease.

# M

**marker:** a button used in older machines to indicate which lead is being recorded.

**midclavicular line:** an anatomical landmark that consists of an imaginary line that runs from the middle of the clavicle down the chest parallel to the arm. (This line is a major reference point on the left side of the body used when examining the heart.)

**\*mitral valve:** the two-cusp valve separating the left atrium from the left ventricle.

**morphology:** shape; the shape of a waveform.

**multifocal PVC:** premature ventricular contractions arising from more than one area of an irritable ventricle.

**\*myocardial infarction:** a heart attack; the death of heart muscle caused by complete blockage of coronary arteries.

**\*myocardium:** the heart muscle.

# N

**non-invasive:** describes procedures which are performed on the body's surface.

**\*normal sinus rhythm (NSR)** or **regular sinus rhythm (RSR):** a heart rhythm that originates in the sinus node and travels down the normal route of the conduction system to the cardiac muscle, resulting in contraction of the heart muscle. On graph paper the rhythm is regular (the beats occur evenly), and the P wave, QRS, and T wave have usual appearances and measurements. The rate is between 60-100 beats per minute.

# P

**\*P wave:** the waveform on the ECG that represents atrial depolarization.

**\*PR interval:** the time period from the onset of the P wave to the beginning of the R wave.

**\*pacemaker rhythm:** an ECG tracing characterized by definite spikes before the P wave and/or QRS which represent the action of an artificial pacemaker.

**pacemaker:** a device that electrically stimulates the heart to cause it to beat.

**parallel:** extending in the same direction and remaining separated by the same distance along the entire length, never crossing paths.

**\*paroxysmal atrial tachycardia:** a rapid burst of tachycardia that comes from an area of the atrium outside of the SA node with present but often difficult to distinguish P waves.

**\*Patient's Bill of Rights:** a document that identifies the basic rights of all patients.

**perfuse:** the forcing of blood into the surrounding tissues and organs by way of the blood vessels.

**\*pericardial sac:** the fibrous covering which completely encloses and protects the heart.

**\*pericarditis:** inflammation of the pericardial sac covering the heart.

**\*Persantine (or dobutamine) stress test:** a procedure used when a patient is unable to physically perform the stress test and the medication, Persantine or dobutamine, is given to the patient in order to artificially raise the heart rate and see how the heart performs when stressed.

**physiology:** the study of the function of the body.

**plaque:** calcified fatty deposits on the inner walls of the arteries of the heart.

**\*polarization:** the period of time when the cellular membrane is in a resting state.

**position control:** the control on the electrocardiograph that adjusts the position of the baseline on the ECG paper.

**posterior wall:** the wall of the heart facing the spine.

**precordial leads:** unipolar or chest leads; used to look at the heart on a horizontal plane from a front to back perspective.

**predisposed:** having an increased risk of developing a disease.

**\*premature atrial contraction (PAC):** an early heart beat that originates in the atria outside of the SA node as a result of atrial irritability.

**\*premature junctional contraction (PJC):** an early heart beat that originates in the AV junctional tissue as a result of irritability and travels retrograde (backward) to the atria and antegrade (forward) to the ventricles.

**\*premature ventricular contraction (PVC):** an early heart beat that originates in the ventricle as a result of ventricular irritability.

**\*prioritize:** to arrange tasks in order of importance.

**protocols:** instructions contained within the software for computerized ECG tests that provide different methods of progressing the speed and incline of the treadmill machine during an ECG stress test.

**\*pulmonary arteries:** large vessels that receive blood from the right ventricle and carry it to the lungs.

**\*pulmonary vein:** one of the two large vessels that returns oxygenated blood from the lungs to the left atrium.

**\*pulmonic valve:** the valve that is in the right ventricle and which separates the ventricle from the pulmonary artery.

**\*Purkinje fibers:** conduction fibers that branch off from the bundle branches and deliver the electrical stimulus to the ventricles, causing the ventricles to contract.

# Q

**\*QRS complex:** a waveform on the ECG that comes after the P wave and represents ventricular depolarization.

# R

**record:** a control on the ECG machine that, when activated, begins the recording of the waveforms onto the graph paper.

**\*refractory period:** the time during repolarization when the cardiac cell cannot respond to another electrical impulse.

**regular:** a heart rhythm in which the beats are evenly spaced.

**\*repolarization:** the period of time when electrolytes move back through the cellular membrane and a resting state is re-established.

**resting state:** the state in which the cardiac cell is not contracting.

**ribs:** a set of 12 pairs of curved bones extending from the spine to the sternum, providing protection to the heart, lungs, and major blood vessels.

**right ventricle:** the lower right chamber of the heart, which receives deoxygenated blood from the right atrium and sends it through the pulmonary valve to the pulmonary arteries.

**\*risk factors:** conditions or states that increase the likelihood of developing a particular disease.

# S

**\*second degree AV heart block (Mobitz Type I):** a disturbance in the electrical activity of the heart that involves a gradual lengthening of the PR interval until a QRS is dropped. Also called Wenckebach.

**\*second degree AV heart block (Mobitz Type II):** a disturbance in the electrical activity of the heart in which an intermittent block between the atrial and ventricular conduction systems results in randomly dropped QRSs and more P waves than QRSs. A high degree of block would result in more blocked QRSs and a slower heart rate.

**segment:** the part of the ECG tracing between two waves.

**\*sensor:** a disc or tab made of plastic that has a metal component as well as a layer or well of gel or conducting substance, and which is placed on a patient's skin in order to pick up electrical activity from the heart where it is transmitted through cables to the ECG machine to be processed. Also called an electrode.

**shortness of breath (SOB):** the feeling of being unable to get enough oxygen; difficulty in breathing; dyspnea.

**sphygmomanometer:** an instrument for measuring blood pressure.

**\*sinoatrial node:** (SA node) the natural pacemaker of the heart, located in the upper part of the right atrium.

**\*sinus arrhythmia:** variation of normal sinus rhythm in which the rhythm is initiated from the sinus node and meets all criteria for NSR except that it is irregular. The rhythm varies with respiration, speeding up with inspiration and slowing with expiration.

**\*sinus bradycardia:** a heart rhythm that originates in the SA node. The rhythm is regular and all waveforms have normal morphology (shape) and duration, but the heart rate is less than 60 bpm.

**sinus rhythm:** a heart rhythm that is produced when the electrical impulse originates from the SA node, creating a very specific waveform shape.

**\*sinus tachycardia:** a heart rhythm that originates in the SA node. The rhythm is regular and all waveforms have normal morphology and duration, but the heart rate is more than 100 bpm.

**standardization button:** a control on the electrocardiograph that makes a mark that should be 10 mm high and 2 mm wide by international agreement. If it is not, then the machine must be recalibrated.

**sternal border:** the edge of the sternum along the outline of the bone.

**sternum:** the breast bone.

**stethoscope:** an instrument used to amplify sound from within the body; the device used to listen for an apical pulse, blood pressure, and bowel or lung sounds.

**\*stylus:** the needle of the ECG machine that forms a tracing on the graph paper.

**\*superior vena cava:** the main vein that drains blood from the upper part of the body into the right atrium of the heart.

**\*supraventricular tachycardia:** a very rapid, relatively regular heart rhythm that originates above the ventricles, either in the AV junction or atria, and is characterized by difficult to distinguish P waves and a possibly widened QRS.

**\*syncopal episode:** a fainting spell.

**\*systole:** the period of time in which the heart muscle is contracting.

# T

**\*T wave:** the waveform on the ECG that represents ventricular repolarization and occurs after the QRS.

**\*tachycardia:** a pulse rate above 100 beats per minute.

**\*target heart rate:** the heart rate an individual should reach to achieve optimal aerobic exertion without chest pain, SOB, or ECG abnormalities.

**\*third degree AV heart block:** a complete block between the atria and the ventricles so that the atria beat independently from the ventricles.

**thrombolytic agents:** medications used to dissolve blood clots.

**\*treadmill stress test:** TMST; a test in which a continuous 12-Lead ECG is recorded during a 15 to 20 minute exercise protocol on a treadmill to determine if heart disease is present; also called stress test, exercise ECG, or simply, treadmill.

**\*tricuspid valve:** the three-cusp valve which controls the flow of blood between the right atrium and right ventricle.

# U

**unipolar lead:** a type of lead for which only a positive sensor is used; the negative sensor exists at an imaginary point created by the positions of the remaining leads.

# V

**valves:** structures in the heart that open in only one direction to ensure the forward movement of the blood.

**vascular:** pertaining to the blood vessels.

**vasodialate:** to expand a blood vessel.

**\*ventricle:** one of the two large muscular pumping chambers of the heart located inferior to the atria.

**ventricular bigeminy:** a pattern consisting of premature ventricular contractions alternating with sinus beats; a heart rhythm in which every other beat is a PVC.

**\*ventricular fibrillation:** a life-threatening condition in which there is no organized atrial or ventricular activity, and the ventricles are quivering and unable to contract.

**\*ventricular hypertrophy:** enlargement of the ventricle.

**\*ventricular tachycardia:** a rapid run of PVCs in a row without any sinus beats.

**ventricular trigeminy:** a heart rhythm consisting of a pattern of premature ventricular contractions occurring every third beat.

**vertical:** perpendicular to a horizontal plane; up and down.

**view:** angle or aspect.

# X

**xiphoid process:** the bony tip of the sternum.


\* denotes key term

# The Manual Alphabet

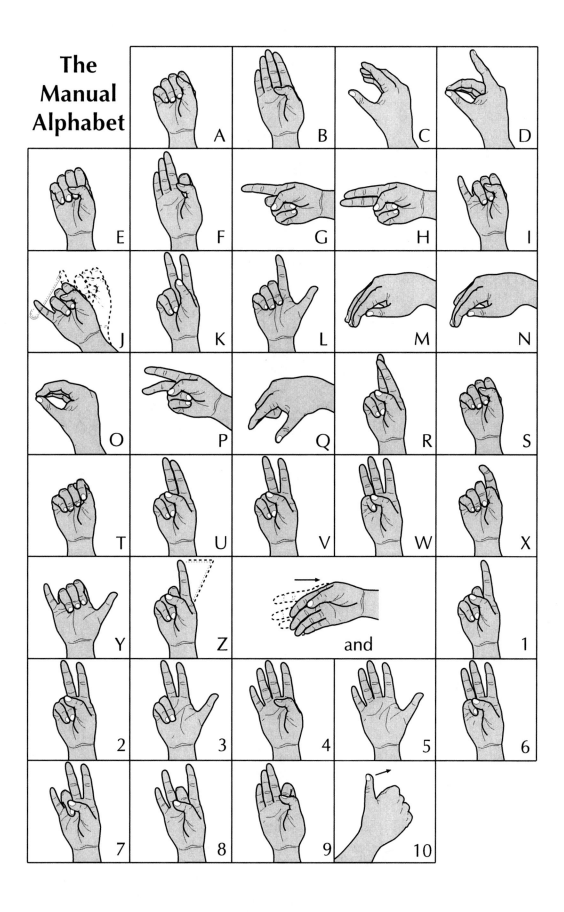

Appendix B-2

# Bibliography

Aehlert, Barbara. *ECG's Made Easy*. Mosby. St. Louis, 1995.

Bonewit-West, Kathy. *Clinical Procedures for Medical Assistants, Fifth Edition*. W.B. Saunders. Philadelphia, 2000.

Burdick Corporation. *Electrocardiography: A Better Way, Second Edition*. Burdick Corporation. Milton, Wisconsin, 1999.

Chabner, Davi-Ellen. *The Language of Medicine, Sixth Edition*. W.B. Saunders. Philadelphia, 2001.

Conover, Mary Boudreau. *Understanding Electrocardiography, Seventh Edition*. Mosby. Portland, 1996.

Copstead, Lee-Ellen C. *Perspectives on Pathophysiology*. W.B. Saunders Company. Philadelphia, 1995.

Crouch, James. *Functional Human Anatomy*. Lea & Febiger. Philadelphia, 1973.

Damjanov, Ivan. *Pathology for the Health-Related Professions*. W.B. Saunders Company. Philadelphia, 1996.

Drew, Barbara J. "Cardiac Rhythm Theory and Analysis," lecture notes. UCSF, 1997.

Ehrat, Karen S. *The Art of Adult and Pediatric EKG Interpretation*. Kendall/Hunt. Dubuque, Iowa, 1985.

Fletcher, Gerald, MD; Balady, Gary, MD; Froelicher, Victor F., MD; Hartley, L. Howard, MD; Haskell, William L., PhD; Pollock, Michael L., PhD. *Exercise Standards, A Statement for Healthcare Professionals From the American Heart Association*. American Heart Association. Dallas, 1995.

Glanze, Walter, ed. *The Mosby Medical Encyclopedia, Revised Edition*. St. Louis: The C.V. Mosby Company, 1992.

Hartshorn, Jeanette; Sole, Mary Lou; Lamborn, Marilyn. *Introduction to Critical Care Nursing, Second Edition.* W.B. Saunders Company. Philadelphia, 1997.

Loeb, Stanley, editor. *Deciphering Difficult ECGs.* Springhouse Corporation. Springhouse, PA, 1983.

Ornish, D.; Brown, S.; Scherwitz, L; and Billlings, J. "Can Lifestyle Changes Reverse Coronary Artery Disease?" *Lancet* 336 (1990): 129-133.

Pagana, Kathleen and Pagana, Timothy. *Mosby's Diagnostic and Laboratory Test Reference, Fourth Edition.* Mosby. St. Louis, 1999.

Robinson, Jean, editor. *Giving Cardiac Care.* Intermed Communications. Springhouse, PA, 1983.

Thomas, Clayton L., MD, MPH. *Taber's Cyclopedic Medical Dictionary, 18th Edition.* Philadelphia: F.A. Davis Company, 1997.

# Index

sphygmomanometers  7-17, 7-18
ST segment  8-14
  depression  7-3, 7-4, 7-22
  elevation  7-3, 7-5, 7-22
sternum  3-3, 5-13
stethoscope  5-13, 7-9, 7-17, 7-18
Streptokinase and Tissue Plasminogen
    Activator (tPA)  2-10
stress  1-7, 1-11, 2-5
  factor 1-11
stylus  5-6
supraventricular tachycardia  9-9 thru 9-10,
    9-18
syncopal episode  6-4, 8-17
systematic rhythm analysis  8-4 thru 8-14
systole  3-14

**T**

T wave  4-4, 8-11, 8-14
tachycardia  6-3, 7-5, 8-18. *See also* sinus
    tachycardia.
target heart rate  7-12
  procedure for determining  7-12 thru 7-13
third degree AV heart block  9-25 thru 9-26
thrombolytic agents  2-10
TMST  7-2. *See* treadmill stress test. *See
    also* treadmill stress test.
  contraindications for  7-6 thru 7-7
  indications for  7-2 thru 7-9
tPA. *See* Streptokinase and Tissue Plasmino-
    gen Activator.
treadmill stress test  1-3, 2-6, 7-2, 7-15
    thru 7-17
tricuspid valve  3-6

**V**

vena cava  3-4
  inferior  3-7
  superior  3-7
ventricles  3-4, 4-4, 8-11, 9-9 thru 9-10
ventricular
  arrhythmias  9-14 thru 9-21
  bigeminy  9-16 thru 9-17
  fibrillation  9-19 thru 9-20
  hypertrophy  5-2
  tachycardia  9-10, 9-18 thru 9-19
  trigeminy  9-16 thru 9-17
voltage  5-12

**W**

wandering baseline  5-36
waveforms  4-3 thru 4-5
  measuring  8-11 thru 8-14
  negative  8-4
  positive  8-4
Wenckebach. *See* second degree AV heart
    block: Mobitz Type I.
William Einthoven  5-5

**X**

xiphoid process  5-13